PROSTATE

&

CANCER

PROSTATE

&

CANCER

A Family Guide to Diagnosis,
Treatment & Survival

FOURTH
EDITION

SHELDON MARKS, M.D.

Da Capo
LIFE
LONG

A MEMBER OF THE PERSEUS BOOKS GROUP

Copyright © 2009 by Sheldon H. F. Marks

Set in 11 point Adobe Garamond by the Perseus Books Group

Cataloging-in-Publication data for this book is available from the Library of Congress.
Library of Congress Control Number: 2002116485
ISBN: 978-0-7382-1347-7
©1995, 1997, 1999, 2003 Sheldon H. F. Marks
Revised 1996, 1997, 1999, 2003, 2009
Published by Da Capo Press
A Member of the Perseus Books Group
www.dacapopress.com

Note: The information in this book is true and complete to the best of our knowledge. This book is intended only as an informative guide for those wishing to know more about health issues. In no way is this book intended to replace, countermand, or conflict with the advice given to you by your own physician. The ultimate decision concerning care should be made between you and your doctor. We strongly recommend you follow his or her advice. Information in this book is general and is offered with no guarantees on the part of the authors or Da Capo Press. The authors and publisher disclaim all liability in connection with the use of this book. The names and identifying details of people associated with events described in this book have been changed. Any similarity to actual persons is coincidental.

Da Capo Press books are available at special discounts for bulk purchases in the United States by corporations, institutions, and other organizations. For more information, please contact the Special Markets Department at the Perseus Books Group, 2300 Chestnut Street, Suite 200, Philadelphia, PA 19103, or call (800) 810-4145, ext. 5000, or e-mail special.markets@perseusbooks.com.

10 9 8 7 6 5

CONTENTS

FOREWORD

I first met Sheldon Marks in the early 1990s and we immediately struck up a friendship. He asked me to write the foreword to the book and I agreed; at that time, I had no idea just how important and informative his book would be. Over the years through the first three editions, countless patients—both my own and those I met at conferences throughout the country—mentioned to me that they had *Prostate & Cancer*. I'm thrilled and honored to be a part of the fourth edition of this outstanding patient-friendly book.

Much has changed since the first edition of this book. Much of the research in prostate cancer has been a result of the U.S. Army's commitment to it, through both the Department of Defense Center for Prostate Disease Research (DoD-CPDR) and the Department of Defense Prostate Cancer Research Program (DoD-PCRP). I served as the director of the DoD-CPDR from its founding in 1991 to the time of my retirement from active duty in 2004. Both of these institutions have contributed a great deal to our current knowledge of prostate cancer; you'll find fruits of this research in this book.

One of the most critical changes has to do with PSA screening. In the early 1990s, we were still in the "Early PSA Era" when the impact of PSA screening wasn't fully known. Up to 20% of men presented with metastatic prostate cancer at first detection! In those "bad old days," it was not uncommon to see men come to us with back pain, leg weakness or even paralysis and soon find out that they were suffering with devastating advanced prostate cancer. Despite hormonal therapy, the prospects for two- to three-year survival were questionable—and five-year survival was rare. Compare this bleak picture with today's more "mature" PSA era when less than 2% of men have metastatic prostate cancer at first detection. This tenfold improvement is due to disease awareness and screening with the PSA blood test.

As I continue my career as the director of the Duke Prostate Center at Duke University Medical Center, I am optimistic and excited about the prostate cancer field. From a treatment perspective, prostate cancer surgery, prostate radiotherapy and prostate cryotherapy are very different now than they were when the first edition of this book was written. Although not perfect, radical prostatectomy is now much less associated with the dreaded complications of incontinence and impotence. Both the minimally invasive open as well as the robotic prostatectomy can be performed by experienced surgeons with much less bleeding, far fewer side effects and much shorter hospitalization than in the past. You'll find out more about these crucial procedures in the following pages. The prostate surgery performed by most urologic oncologists is far different today than in the not-so-distant past. Similar comments can be said of other techniques that have been vastly improved through better equipment and greater experience. There are other advancements you'll discover in these pages. Procedures such as high intensity focused ultrasound (HIFU) are on the horizon, as are better strategies for "focal therapy," and Dr. Marks addresses crucial questions about these. There have also been multiple advancements in medications; herein you'll find information about the latest FDA-approved treatments. The field is continuing to change and evolve; here, Dr. Marks gives you the most up-to-date information to help you and your loved ones make the best, most informed decisions regarding your health care.

Thanks to Dr. Sheldon Marks and his tireless efforts, patients and loved ones have a clear, concise and thorough resource. For men and their families facing a diagnosis of prostate cancer, *Prostate & Cancer* is invaluable.

JUDD W. MOUL, M.D., FACS
Professor of Surgery and Chief, Urologic Surgery
Director, Duke Prostate Center
Duke University Medical Center

ACKNOWLEDGMENTS

Thanks to all of my friends and colleagues who continually inspire and support me as this book evolves. Special thanks to my patients, their wives and families, who openly share their experiences so that together we can empower other patients to take control of their health care decisions by educating them. Thank you to all of the renowned experts who have given their time and reviewed every edition and shared their insights and wisdom so that this can truly be the ultimate resource on prostate cancer. Special thanks also to Brenda Malone Marks, who was instrumental in concept, development and writing the first three editions of this book.

Most importantly, I wish to thank my family. I thank my parents for being the role models they are—my late mother who fought ovarian cancer with grace and class for eight and a half years, and my father who has shown me through example how to achieve anything; I thank my children, Matthew, Jordan and Ally, for giving my life true meaning; and I thank Page—my wife, who remains an inspiration and continuously shows me that no matter what, the glass is always half full.

DEDICATION

This book is dedicated to all the men and their families who courageously live the fight every day against their prostate cancer. Only they understand the battles that must be fought to win the war.

I also dedicate this book to the tireless efforts of all the men and women in research labs around the world who have dedicated their lives to finding new answers to the questions about prostate cancer, its prevention and its cures.

PREFACE

Prostate cancer continues to be a highly visible public cancer, often mentioned with the diagnosis of elected officials and celebrities. As more public figures have announced that they have cancer of the prostate, it has become a frequent news item and topic of discussion in many households throughout the country.

Prostate cancer has touched the lives of high-profile people such as presidential candidates Rudy Giuliani and John Kerry; golfer Arnold Palmer; Senators Bob Dole, Ted Stevens, Richard Shelby and William Roth; General Norman Schwarzkopf; Colin Powell and actors and entertainers such as Bill Bixby, Telly Savalas and Frank Zappa, to name a few.

More than 186,320 men were diagnosed with prostate cancer in 2008, and more than 28,660 men previously diagnosed will die as a result of it in 2008. Prostate cancer has become the most-diagnosed non-skin cancer in America and the second-leading killer of men. Articles appear in national magazines, questions are called in on radio talk shows and newspapers frequently report a new idea or breakthrough in the field of prostate cancer.

It seems the more we hear and read, the more confused we become. Even many primary-care doctors seem confused about whether prostate cancer is a significant disease and which treatment options are best, if any.

I believe that the fear of the unknown is the most overwhelming and traumatic result of all the confusion about this disease. Unfortunately, short of spending an hour or two in personal consultation with a urologist, there is really no complete and accurate source of information available.

There are numerous books on prostate disease in general, or on men's health, usually with a chapter on prostate cancer. These books often tell you what the author thinks you should know about prostate cancer. But the topic of prostate cancer is too important and too controversial to confine its discussion to just a few pages. There are many books about prostate cancer, but many of the patient's real questions are left unanswered. When the first edition of *Prostate & Cancer* came out in 1995, no one had any idea how much this book would be accepted and used around the world. Since then, many dozens of books have been written, often using the format or even pieces of this book. Yet none really seem to be as effective as this. In this fourth edition, I continue focusing on the questions and concerns that real people have. Too many books come across like lectures, often quoting confusing and unnecessary statistics and numbers. Others are simply personal accounts and opinions.

As the men's health expert for WebMD for more than five years, I have continued to answer questions and calm readers' fears through education and understandable facts.

Many of us will spend months researching a new car or weeks reading up on the latest lawn mower. But when it comes to our health and our bodies, many of us, especially men, are satisfied with a five-minute explanation of the problem. Some men will accept the doctor's recommendations without question. The choices we make will definitely impact on the quality of our remaining years and very possibly the length of our lives.

You have a right to understand exactly what is going on with your body, the treatment options you have and the long-term impact of the decisions you make about your care. This book will educate you and answer your questions about your prostate and cancer. It will give you what you need to be an informed consumer. It will enable you to take control and make the best decisions about your future that will affect your health and well-being.

Prostate & Cancer is intended to serve as a resource to give you a foundation for informed discussion about your health with your doctor. This book is not intended to replace your physician, who can individualize your particular situation while considering other factors, such as your general health, your family longevity and the specifics of your problem.

At my patients' suggestion and urging, I have taken my notes and expanded them into this book to provide the basic information necessary for an individual to make an informed decision regarding the evaluation and treatment of prostate cancer.

This book can't possibly cover all the details specific to you. Likewise, there is no way you should make decisions regarding your health based solely on my comments here. This book is written from my own personal experiences and is not intended as a comprehensive resource on the subjects. It contains my interpretation of current philosophies and controversies regarding cancer of the prostate. I have also brought together the latest ideas and cutting-edge research from world-class specialists, professional meetings and journals. This book is to be used to stimulate intelligent discussions and conversation with your doctors, and to get you to ask questions and seek out more information on the topics relevant to you.

The continued worldwide demand and positive feedback from physicians, nurses, patients and their families has led us to produce this updated and re-vised edition.

I wrote this book to empower and educate men and their families with questions about prostate cancer. If this book was given to you, please thank the friend, doctor or company that made it possible. Only through positive feedback will they continue to distribute and sponsor this book and other educational resources. If you have any thoughts or suggestions, we encourage you to let us know.

It is my sincerest hope that this book will answer many of your questions and thereby ease your fears so you can be your own best health advocate.

Knowledge is power.

SHELDON H.F. MARKS, M.D.
850 North Kolb Road
Tucson, Arizona 85710

Adjunct Assistant Professor
Department of Urology
Tufts University School of Medicine
Boston, Massachusetts

Clinical Associate Professor
Division of Urology
Department of Surgery
University of Arizona College of Medicine
Tucson, Arizona

ANATOMY AND FUNCTION OF THE PROSTATE GLAND

T he prostate gland, essential for reproduction, is one of those body parts that a man rarely thinks about—that is, until he begins to have problems or concerns. Over time and under the influence of normal male hormones, the prostate can enlarge or develop cancer.

To understand prostate disease and its impact, it is important to have a general understanding of the normal pelvic and genitourinary anatomy that are involved.

The function of the prostate gland is to add vital nutrients and fluid to the sperm. The prostate is a relatively small, walnut-sized gland that sits just below the *urinary bladder* in the bottom of the pelvis, surrounding the *urethra*. It is this position that can lead to difficulties later in life. As the gland enlarges from normal growth or from cancer, it can squeeze down on the urinary passage and make it increasingly difficult to urinate.

When fathering children is no longer a goal, the prostate no longer serves its main purpose.

When fathering children is no longer a goal, the prostate no longer serves its main purpose. However, the gland remains, and in the presence of normal

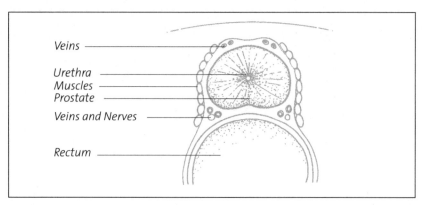

PROSTATE CANCER CROSS-SECTION. Cross-section of prostate gland shows location of nerves and blood vessels, as well as prostate position next to rectal wall.

male hormones, the prostate continues to grow until at some point it may cause problems.

The prostate gland is actually a collection of tiny glands that secrete fluid encased as one organ. The outside of the prostate is surrounded by a thin capsule of compressed fibrous tissue. Outside the prostate is a layer of fat.

Behind the prostate, just a few millimeters away, is the front wall of the rectum. On each side of the gland are nerves and blood vessels. These nerves are all-important when we address the treatment choices for prostate cancer and problems that can occur.

The prostate is divided into right and left sides, called *lobes.* The tip of the prostate farthest from the bladder is the *apex.* The wider portion next to the bladder is the *base.* The front is called *anterior,* and the rear *posterior.*

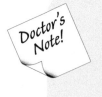

Over the years it has become clear to me that most men have absolutely no idea what their prostate is or where it is located. One of my patients, a retired engineer, had obviously done extensive reading before he visited my office. He was proud that he knew so much about his prostate. That is, until he asked me what the prostate did for women and why women didn't have prostate problems. . . . Sometimes a little information is just that, a little information.

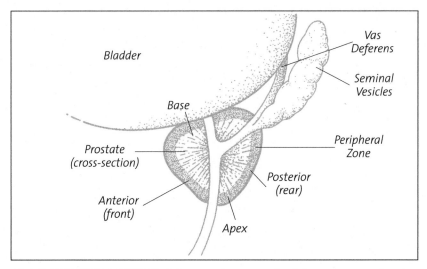

PROSTATE DESCRIPTION. Side view of prostate gland shows terms used to describe the top (base), bottom (apex), front (anterior) and back (posterior).

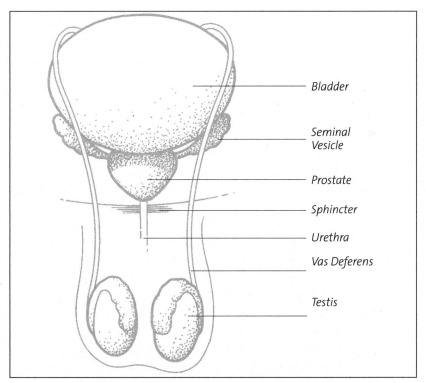

PELVIC ANATOMY. Prostate is located immediately below the bladder in the pelvis. Seminal vesicles and the vas deferens from both testicles drain into the prostate.

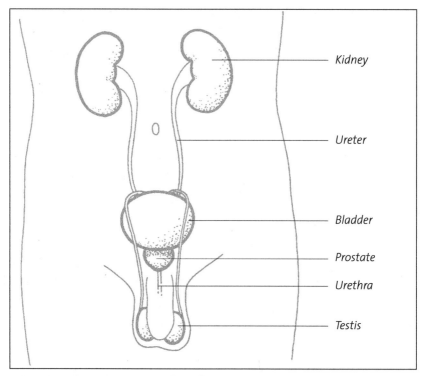

Kidney

Ureter

Bladder

Prostate

Urethra

Testis

UROGENITAL ANATOMY. Kidneys filter the blood and drain urine down the ureters into the bladder. Here it is stored before coming out the urethra, through the prostate.

The *vas deferens* is the tube that leads the sperm from the testicles and empties into the urethra inside the prostate. Fluid from adjacent glands called the *seminal vesicles* also drains into the prostate. These glands are next to the prostate and below the bladder. The testicles not only make the sperm but also produce the male hormone *testosterone*, which is delivered directly into the bloodstream. (See illustration above.)

The bladder sits above the prostate, in the bottom of the pelvis. It serves two purposes. First, the bladder is a container, or reservoir, for urine, so you can build up urine and empty when you choose to, rather than when it is created. The second function is to serve as the muscle that squeezes out the urine when given the necessary messages from your brain. Urine is made in the kidneys by filtering waste products from the blood. The urine then drains down the ureters into the bladder.

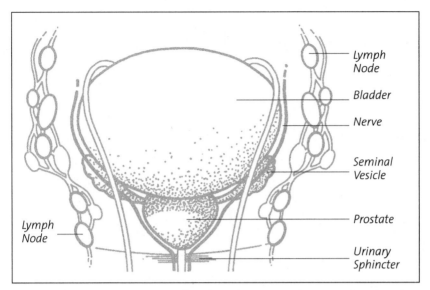

LYMPH DRAINAGE. Lymphatic fluid from the prostate drains into lymph nodes on both sides of the pelvis. Cancer in the prostate can follow this pathway and spread to these lymph nodes.

The urethra is the tube that leads from the bladder through the prostate, past the *urinary sphincter* and out the penis to the opening, called the *urethral meatus.*

The urinary sphincter, a collection of circular muscle fibers just below the prostate, helps to prevent leakage of urine when you cough, move or are physically active. Much of the control (called *continence*) of urine actually occurs at the bladder *neck*. There, all of the circular muscle fibers come together like a funnel.

Veins of the prostate drain blood out and up toward the heart alongside the spinal column. The *lymphatics* drain from the prostate to a number of small *lymph nodes* clustered along the wall of the pelvis on both sides.

What is the lymphatic system?

The lymphatics serve as the cleaning system for the body. All cells of the body are bathed by lymph fluid—clear, slippery fluid that sometimes oozes from scrapes or abrasions. This fluid is filtered through lymph nodes, where

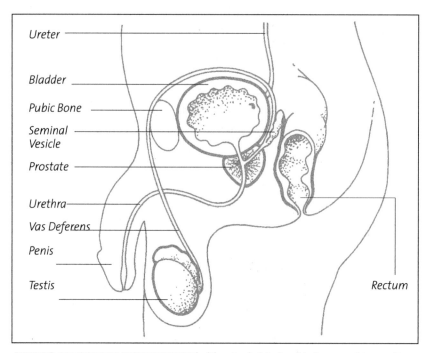

Ureter

Bladder

Pubic Bone

Seminal
Vesicle

Prostate

Urethra

Vas Deferens

Penis

Testis

Rectum

PELVIC ANATOMY, SIDE VIEW. Bladder sits behind pubic bone and immediately in front of rectum. Prostate gland is below bladder and surrounds urethra just as it leaves the bladder.

any impurities, germs or cancer cells are captured. The filtered lymph fluid then flows back into the bloodstream.

Noncancerous Prostate Enlargement (BPH)

For reasons still unclear, the prostate in most men slowly grows and increases in size. This growth, called *benign prostatic hyperplasia*, or *BPH*, is not cancerous. It can, however, seriously impact on a man's quality of life by causing blockage to the urine flow. This can result in a number of annoying and bothersome symptoms, such as frequent daytime and nighttime urination, dribbling and difficulty starting and stopping the urinary stream. (See the list of symptoms on page 38.)

For years, treatment options for BPH were limited. Most men who had the problem ultimately had surgery. During the past decade, however, new breakthroughs and advances have provided a wide range of options that can

Does having an enlarged prostate increase my odds of getting prostate cancer?

Having enlargement of the prostate (BPH) does not increase your risks for developing prostate cancer.

often reduce the symptoms without the risks and potential side effects of surgery.

Do I need treatment if my prostate is enlarged but I don't have any problems urinating?

No, not usually. Unless your prostate is causing real problems with your bladder from incomplete emptying, infections or bleeding, you don't need any treatment.

What are the options for treating the symptoms of an enlarged prostate?

There are five basic options, each with definite advantages and disadvantages:
1. Doing nothing
2. Taking alpha-blocker medication (Hytrin, Cardura Flomax, Uroxatral or Rapaflo
3. Taking a 5 alpha reductase inhibitor (Proscar, Avodart) or saw palmetto
4. Having minimally invasive therapy—laser surgery, vaporization, thermal or microwave therapy
5. Having a standard surgical resection of the prostate

How is doing nothing a treatment choice?

You can always choose not to treat your symptoms. If you are not bothered much by blockage symptoms, then it may be reasonable just to watch and wait. You may find that you are doing better, staying the same or getting worse. Of course, if the symptoms do become a problem for you, then you should talk to your doctor about your other choices.

It is always interesting to talk to two men who have the same urinating problems. One may be miserable getting up twice each night to urinate, while the other is thrilled that he's not getting up more often.

What is an alpha-blocker?

This type of medication was originally used only for the treatment of high blood pressure. We knew this medication worked by relaxing a very specific type of muscle fiber found in the walls of blood vessels. We soon learned that these muscles are also found around the prostate and bladder base. When these muscles contract, they squeeze the urethra shut and can cause the annoying symptoms often associated with an enlarged prostate. When these muscles are relaxed by taking an alpha-blocker every day, the urethra and prostate open up. This can result in a rapid and dramatic improvement in urination.

What are the names of these alpha-blockers?

Hytrin (terazosin), Cardura (doxazosin), Uroxatral (alfuzosin) and Flomax (tamsulosin) are commonly used alpha-blockers for the symptoms of blockage. A brand-new medication, Rapaflo (silodosin), was released at the end of 2008.

The use of alpha-blockers over the past few years has eliminated the need for surgery for many men.

Do alpha-blockers work for most men?

The good news is that most men who try these medications will see a dramatic improvement in their urination, with a reduction of their annoying symptoms. This usually happens within a few weeks. I have been very impressed with how well most of my patients respond in a short time. A small number may not tolerate the medication or may not experience an improvement.

Does taking alpha-blockers for my prostate protect me from getting prostate cancer?

No. These are excellent medications to relax the muscles that squeeze the prostate, thus improving urination. For many men, these medications may eliminate the need for surgery. Taking them does absolutely nothing to reduce your risks of developing prostate cancer.

Are there any side effects from taking alpha-blockers?
In the first few days on the medication, some men may experience dizziness, light-headedness or fatigue, and on very rare occasions may faint. This can be prevented if you stand up slowly during the first few days as your body adapts to the medication. I mention this only as a precautionary note. These symptoms are less of a problem with Flomax, Rapaflo and Uroxatral, which are more selective third-generation alpha-blockers.

Do alpha-blockers interact with other medications?
Because these medications can also lower high blood pressure, it is important for you to coordinate with your primary-care physician or cardiologist, especially if you are already taking other medications for high blood pressure. Flomax and Uroxatral do not usually affect blood pressure. If you take a medication for erectile dysfunction, you should check with your doctor because the combination can cause a dangerous drop in blood pressure.

How do Proscar and Avodart work?
Proscar (finasteride) and Avodart (dutasteride), called 5 alpha reductase inhibitors, work by blocking the normal formation of male hormone byproduct in the prostate. This byproduct, called *DHT*, is a very powerful stimulator of prostate growth, far more powerful than testosterone. When DHT is blocked, the prostate may shrink in size and this shrinking can improve urination. As with alpha-blockers, if Proscar or Avodart are successful, you will need to take the medication daily as long as you want to have the benefits.

Does taking Proscar or Avodart reduce my risks for getting prostate cancer?
Studies suggest that yes, if you are at risk for prostate cancer, taking either of these medications can prevent prostate cancer development.

What are the side effects of Proscar or Avodart?
The side effects of Proscar or Avodart are primarily sexual, with about 4% of men describing impotence and less than 4% complaining of a reduced sex interest.

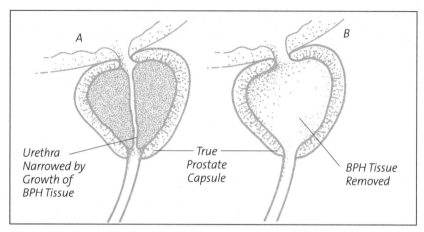

NONCANCEROUS PROSTATE TISSUE. A. Noncancerous prostate tissue (BPH) grows and compresses the urethra, resulting in urination difficulty. B. Following transurethral resection of the prostate (TURP), this nonmalignant tissue is removed, leaving the prostate capsule intact.

What are the benefits of taking Proscar or Avodart?

Proscar and Avodart have been shown to prevent serious complications and urinary retention as well as reduce the need for surgery for men with enlarged prostates. This is especially true if the prostate specific antigen (PSA) is greater than 1.7 or the prostate is larger than 30 cc (golf-ball size).

Can taking Proscar or Avodart cause problems?

There are some concerns that Proscar or Avodart may confuse the interpretation of the PSA level. This is because Proscar and Avodart can reduce PSA levels (see Chapter 6)—sometimes drastically—from 10% to 90% of what they actually are.

How does laser surgery work?

The urologist can use a laser to destroy the prostate tissue that is causing blockage. A laser is pointed into or placed in the tissue through the urethra. Usually performed under anesthesia, this operation can be performed as an outpatient procedure. The patient can return to work or normal activities the next day. The laser surgery is safe for on patients who are taking Coumadin (warfarin).

Are there any problems with laser surgery?
This is one of many treatment options; urologists are learning exactly what technique works best for each patient. Only time will tell if laser surgery is as effective as more standard surgery. Personally, I am very happy with results for the men I have treated with the laser. In the past it was my preferred treatment for prostate obstruction.

How is an enlarged prostate surgically treated?
The standard treatment for many years was always the *TURP*, or *transurethral resection of the prostate*. This operation is performed under anesthesia through a fiber-optic instrument. It requires no incision, and is very well tolerated with rapid recovery. A TURP is the gold standard against which all other treatments are compared.

Looking through the instrument that is placed up the penis, the prostate tissue that is causing the blockage can be seen. It is this tissue that is literally scooped out with the instrument, leaving only the shell of the prostate remaining. For very large prostate glands, urologists sometimes perform an operation through an incision in the lower abdomen (open prostatectomy), but this technique is less common. The tissue removed is examined to be sure no cancer is present.

Does having my prostate opened up with a TURP mean I don't have to worry about getting prostate cancer?
No. Even though the tissue causing the blockage has been removed, you are still at risk of developing prostate cancer in the rim of tissue left behind. You must get an annual evaluation and PSA blood test to be sure no cancer develops.

Do the pathologists examine for cancer all the pieces of the prostate tissue removed during the TURP procedure?
No, they look at a representative sample of the tissue provided. It is almost impossible and too expensive for pathologists to analyze every piece of prostate tissue. If they look at a good percentage of the tissue, they will have a fairly good idea of how much and what kind of cancer is present, if any.

What other ways can my prostate be treated?

There are many new "minimally invasive" techniques, including hyperthermia, microwave therapy, needle ablation, ultrasound and vaporization. Each technique has advantages and disadvantages. Most are not as effective as a TURP, but have fewer risks. The new microwave therapies involve simply placing a special catheter in the urethra for about one hour, under mild sedation, in the office. You avoid the risks of surgery and anesthesia.

PROSTATE CANCER 2

P rostate cancer is just one of literally hundreds of different types of cancers that can develop in the human body. Though each cancer is different, all cancers have certain similarities. Prostate cancer has a number of unique aspects. Before we can address prostate cancer, we need to review cancer in general, including its growth and causes.

What is cancer?

Cancer is a multistep process of *disordered and abnormal cell growth*. It is a disease of cell structure and function. Within each individual cell, thousands of microscopic *tubules* serve as a skeleton to the cell (see diagram on next page). The tubules serve as the connection between cells as well.

Tubules provide the way for cells to "communicate," or work and function with each other. With cancer, these tubules are distorted so that cells no longer function as they were intended. They no longer communicate with each other.

Normal cells have certain limits to their growth as they contact cells around them. With the tubule mechanism lost, cells continue to grow without controls. They are no longer limited by normal patterns of growth.

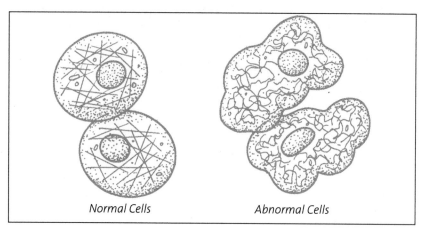

Normal Cells　　　　　　Abnormal Cells

CELL STRUCTURE. Normal body cells have an organized and regular skeleton made up of microscopic tubules that allow for normal growth. Cancer cells have lost this organized pattern, with distortion of the normal microtubules and loss of the normal cell shape and growth patterns.

Most cells have a certain predetermined or "programmed" life span. Normal programmed cell death or cellular self-destruction is called *apoptosis*. With cancer, this can be altered. The cells not only grow beyond their normal borders, but they also do not die when they should. Normal cell growth slows down toward the end of the life cycle (senescence). Cancer cells fail to do this.

Simply, cancer cells grow without the usual controls and limits. They keep growing well beyond their normal boundaries and can spread into other tissues of the body.

What is a malignancy?
A malignancy is a cancerous growth that has the potential to spread and cause injury or death.

Are all cancers the same?
No. There are hundreds of types of cancer. Each type of tissue and cell can lose the ability to grow normally. Some are slow growing; others, fast. Each one has different growth patterns, properties and characteristics. Each has weaknesses that we hope to identify and take advantage of with treatment—

Is cancer contagious?

No. Cancer is an internal cellular abnormality that starts within the cells of an individual. One person cannot "catch" a cancer from another. Cancer cannot be spread like a virus or bacteria.

whether surgery, radiation, chemotherapy, hormone therapy or some of the new immune therapies.

Does cancer always cause death?

No. Some types of cancers are almost always life threatening, while others will rarely lead to death. Most cancers are somewhere in the middle. Prostate cancer can be slow growing and of minimal concern, or it can grow rapidly, spread and possibly lead to death. Sometimes prostate cancer starts as slow growing and evolves into fast growing. We use the term *aggressive* to refer to these fast-growing, potentially life-threatening cancers.

What causes cancers to grow?

Cancers develop for a variety of reasons. Cancer is a genetic-environmental interaction. Sometimes we know what can stimulate a cancer to start growing. Smoking, for example, can cause irritation, which can lead to lung cancer. With many other types of cancer, researchers have no idea what starts the cancer's growth from otherwise normal cells.

We know that many environmental chemicals and substances can initiate or stimulate cancer growth. Research now points strongly to a person's diet—especially a high-fat, low-fiber diet over many years—as a contributing factor to many cancers.

Genetics is involved as well. Some cancers seem to run in families. Scientists have identified certain genetic weaknesses that can be passed on by parents. In certain situations, these weaknesses can enable cancers to grow.

New cancer growth is a combination of the overproduction of cancer stimulants and reduced amounts of cancer growth blockers (inhibitors). Cigarette smoking is linked to more aggressive prostate cancers.

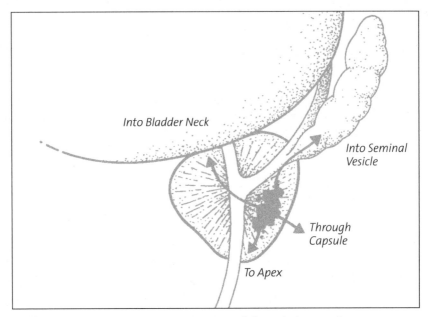

Into Bladder Neck

Into Seminal Vesicle

Through Capsule

To Apex

CANCER SPREAD. Prostate cancer can spread through the capsule into surrounding tissues and the bladder neck, through the apex or into the adjacent seminal vesicles.

How does cancer spread?

As cancers grow, they begin to stimulate the growth of new blood vessels.
These new vessels are known to be leaky. The cells of the cancer squeeze
through the microscopic gaps and get into the bloodstream. Cancer cells
then travel along with the blood throughout the body. When the cells find
an environment that encourages growth, they can settle in and grow. This
growth of cancer cells away from the main cancer is called *metastasis*. As the
cancer cells start to grow, they stimulate the abnormal growth of new blood
vessels (*angiogenesis*). Angiogenesis is normally activated only in wound healing. These new blood vessels provide the nutrients needed for the cancer to
establish itself, grow and spread. Cancer cannot grow more than 2 mm without new blood vessels! Prostate cancer is angiogenesis dependent. Without
new blood vessels, prostate cancer cannot survive. Researchers are looking at
ways of controlling the spread of cancer by blocking angiogenesis.

What is prostate cancer?

Prostate cancer is a malignant growth of the glandular cells within the prostate. Normally these cells are located in the glands that produce the fluid that makes up most of the semen. But, under certain circumstances, these cells can lose their normal controls and start to grow out of control, becoming cancerous. These malignant cells lose their natural surrounding layers that are a barrier to spread.

How does prostate cancer start?

Like all cancers, it probably starts as a tiny change in just a few cells. Over many years, perhaps even 20 or more, this can develop into a tiny cluster that gradually enlarges. As the cancer grows, it gains momentum, growing faster.

How fast does prostate cancer grow?

In most situations, prostate cancer grows very slowly over many years, perhaps even decades. But it eventually grows faster and gets larger. Some prostate cancers may grow very rapidly and can be quite deadly.

What stimulates prostate cancer to grow?

Prostate cancer is in a class of cancers, like breast cancer, that is *hormone-sensitive*. In the prostate, the hormone *testosterone* is converted into another very powerful hormone, DHT. In prostate cancer, these hormones stimulate the cancer cells' uncontrolled growth.

What happens when prostate cancer spreads?

As the cancer grows, it invades surrounding tissues. The cancer then stimulates new nerves to grow, and then the cancer travels alongside these small nerves to outer layers. At first, it just grows into more and more of the prostate. When the cancer reaches the outside capsule or shell of the prostate gland, the cancer can grow through it into the fat surrounding the prostate. Cancer can also grow into the adjacent bladder or the seminal vesicles.

Where else in the body does prostate cancer spread?

Prostate cancer spreads to two main areas of the body. One, to the lymph nodes that drain the prostate, and second, to the bone, mostly of the spine

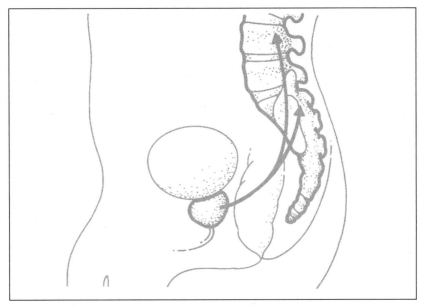

CANCER SPREAD TO THE SPINE. Prostate-cancer cells can spread up through the veins that drain the prostate from the pelvis, alongside and into the bones of the spine.

and ribs. Specifically, the cancer grows inside the bone marrow, which is the inside of the bone where active growth of new bone takes place.

Why does prostate cancer spread to the spine?
Cancer cells leave the prostate in the bloodstream. As the blood leaves the prostate gland, it travels through a web of veins alongside the prostate and into the spine. The blood then passes into the bones of the spinal column. Prostate-cancer cells grow here because it is the first body environment the cells encounter that encourages their growth.

What are the causes of prostate cancer?
We really don't know what causes prostate cancer. Researchers around the world are investigating causes now. It may be years before we have any definitive answers. However, recent evidence suggests that prostate cancers may develop because of genetic imbalances, which can lead to mutations over time. These imbalances may be accelerated by environmental factors such as diet.

We know some genes in every cell in the body prevent cancer by blocking or suppressing cancerous changes in the tissues. When these preventive genes are blocked, there's nothing to keep the cancer from starting up and growing. There are also genes that lie dormant, but under yet-unknown circumstances they activate and stimulate cancer-cell growth. It appears as if all these factors may play some role.

Is it true that most prostate cancers being detected today are really insignificant and should be ignored?

Absolutely not. Almost 30,000 men die each year from prostate cancer in the United States alone. Reviews of patients who have been treated with surgery show that if the cancer is big enough to be detected with modern techniques, it is most often large enough to be a threat to the person's life. It should not be ignored. Truly insignificant cancers are rarely detected.

Why is there controversy about whether or not to detect or treat prostate cancer?

Prostate cancer is a disease in which growth and treatments are measured in ten to twenty years or more. The final answers about advances in diagnosis and treatment can take quite a long time. In fact, only recently have studies shown the definite and significant benefits of early detection and treatment. One must always remember that these studies are good at predicting results for a large number of men, but are poor at telling a specific individual what he should or shouldn't do. Many studies are flawed because they only look at results of studies over just five or seven years. Clearly, if the cancer is a disease of ten to fifteen years or more, then labeling a treatment as a success or failure at five years out is not really helpful.

Does having a vasectomy increase my risks of getting cancer?

No. Only one of several studies suggests there may be a relationship between men who have had a vasectomy and whether or not they are diagnosed with prostate cancer many years later. Many recent studies don't show any increased risks if you have had a vasectomy.

Urologists are fairly certain that this correlation is simply a statistical co-incidence. It is important to remember that vasectomy and prostate cancer do not appear to be cause and effect.

Does ultraviolet radiation from the sun have anything to do with prostate cancer?

Some studies show that as the exposure to ultraviolet (UV) light goes up (meaning more sun exposure), the rates of prostate cancer go down. Researchers believe that the increased sun exposure raises the body's own natural vitamin D, which helps to reduce prostate-cancer risks. Men in parts of the world that have less sun have higher rates of prostate cancer.

What about exposure to chemicals at work? Does this increase risk?

Certain occupational hazards may play a role, but this relationship is still very weak. Men who work in rubber factories or with certain chemicals, such as cadmium, as well as farmers, seem to have an increased risk. For the farmers, it may be exposure to pesticides and other industrial chemicals, or perhaps it's the high-fat diet many eat.

Why do we know so little about cancer of the prostate?

There are five reasons to explain why doctors and researchers know as little as we do about such an important cancer.

1. There has never been very much money invested in prostate-cancer research.
2. Prostate cancer takes so long to grow and progress (decades) that short-term studies really aren't of much use. Long-term studies are difficult to start up and keep going. By the time the study is long enough, the treatments are different.
3. The disease is different from person to person, and each variant of the disease behaves differently. It is almost impossible to compare one treatment with another.
4. Scientists, researchers and physicians have a relatively poor understanding the basic mechanisms of prostate-cancer growth and spread.

5. Most of the research that has been done has been inadequate, often
    with serious errors that put the results in question.

Although we do know quite a lot about prostate cancer from clinical experience, we are now seeing significant scientific studies being funded. We
hope these studies will give us valuable information in the future about treatment and the disease itself. I encourage you to be vocal with your congres-
sional representatives by asking for more funding and support for
prostate-cancer research. Whether we can make a difference in our own lives
remains to be seen, but we can definitely make a difference for our children
and our grandchildren.

Do all prostate cancers grow the same?

No, not at all. Many prostate cancers may look similar at any given point,
comparing one man with another, but the cancers may have different rates
of growth. One may grow very fast, not responding at all to treatments, while
another cancer that appears to be the same might grow slowly.

Who's at risk?

All men are potentially at risk of developing prostate cancer at some point
in their lifetime. As the population grows older, more prostate cancer is going
to be detected. This is most often a disease of older men. However, young
men can get and die from prostate cancer as well. As modern medicine continues to keep us living longer and healthier lives, many of us will eventually
be diagnosed with prostate cancer. In other words, if you live long enough,

Is there any way to tell which cancers may become deadly and
which will grow slowly and probably not affect my life span?

There is no way to accurately tell which cancers will become
deadly. Until there is, most doctors believe it is appropriate
for young, healthy men to pursue age-appropriate aggressive
therapy.

> *Does having a relative with prostate cancer increase my risk?*
>
> **?**
>
> Certain groups of men are more likely to be diagnosed with prostate cancer. We know from recent studies that if there are any males in your family with prostate cancer, your risk for developing the disease is higher.
>
> The younger the family member is when he's diagnosed with prostate cancer, the higher the risks that other male relatives will be diagnosed with prostate cancer at a younger age. If you have any female relatives with breast or ovarian cancer, your risks for prostate cancer are also increased.

sooner or later you will probably develop prostate cancer. Whether or not the cancer will affect your quality of life or longevity is a different issue.

Does it make a difference where I live in the United States?
Yes, studies show that there is a higher death rate from prostate cancer in the Northwest, the Rocky Mountain states, the north-central United States, New England and South Atlantic areas.

Are my sons at risk of developing prostate cancer?
Yes, there is an increased risk for all male relatives. This includes your sons, brothers, cousins and nephews. They should all be seen yearly for the PSA and exam, starting at age 40, and should make preventive dietary changes now. I have heard so many times of men who warned their relatives, and they were subsequently found to have cancer at an early stage.

Does my father's being diagnosed at age 52 increase my risk much?
Yes. The younger the relative is when he is diagnosed with prostate cancer, the higher the risk that you may develop prostate cancer as well.

Does that mean I might get prostate cancer when I'm young too?
Your odds of developing prostate cancer also at a young age are definitely increased. In this situation, prevention and early detection are most important.

At age 42, one of my patients was diagnosed with prostate cancer. He had no family history of any cancer. His older brothers were naturally at increased risk. Yet when they went to their doctors for a PSA and digital rectal exam, they were both told it was not necessary until they turned 50. This was one of those unfortunate situations where the doctor remembered only part of the recommendations. Subsequent evaluation showed the brothers were fine. They will continue their annual checkups, with doctors who understand their increased risks.

Is it true African American men are more likely to get prostate cancer?

For reasons we still don't understand, black men are more likely to get prostate cancer at a younger age, and often with a more aggressive strain. In fact, black American men have the highest rate of prostate cancer of any population or group anywhere in the world. Survival is the same when young black men opt for surgical removal of the cancer. Early detection is the key. Research suggests that a high-fat diet and reduced sun exposure may play a

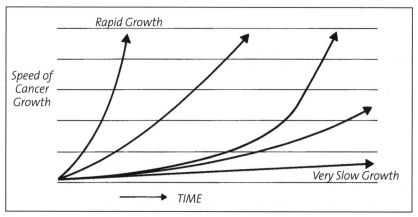

CANCER GROWTH RATES. Prostate-cancer growth can be unpredictable. For some men it can grow very slowly throughout their lives, or very rapidly, resulting in death, or any pattern in between.

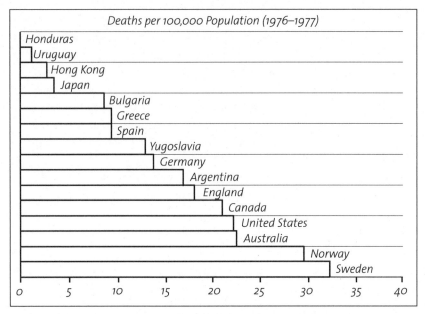

Deaths per 100,000 Population (1976–1977)

Honduras
Uruguay
Hong Kong
Japan
Bulgaria
Greece
Spain
Yugoslavia
Germany
Argentina
England
Canada
United States
Australia
Norway
Sweden

0   5   10   15   20   25   30   35   40

PROSTATE-CANCER DEATH RATES AROUND THE WORLD. Prostate-cancer deaths are highest per person in Scandinavia. They are lowest in the Far East and Central America. Chart courtesy American Cancer Society 1999.

role. Other ethnic groups may have less risk, including those men with Asian ancestry.

Is prostate cancer contagious? Can my wife catch cancer by having sex with me if I have prostate cancer?
No, you cannot catch prostate cancer or any cancer from someone else. Cancer is a process in which the cells of your body lose their self-controlling ability. This process cannot affect another person through contact, sexual relations or living in close quarters.

What are the official recommendations of the American Cancer Society?
All men age 50 and over should have an annual digital rectal exam and PSA blood test. The PSA test is explained in detail in Chapter 6.

Men with a family history of prostate cancer should get an annual PSA test and digital rectal exam starting at age 40.

Hereditary prostate cancer is a concern to all related males, especially when the cancer is discovered early in life. African Americans should have an annual digital rectal exam and PSA test starting at age 40.

> **CANCER TREATMENT GOALS**
> Reduce number of men who develop cancer
> Improve early detection
> Improve treatments

What can I do now?
The key to a healthy and normal life is early detection and appropriate treatment. Eat a diet high in fresh fruit and vegetables and fresh herbs and low in fat from red meat and dairy.

DIET AND NUTRITION— THE EFFECT ON PROSTATE CANCER

3

O ver the past few years, more and more research has demonstrated the strong association between diet and cancer, a connection that was initially considered "fringe" thinking. Today most major academic and cancer institutions have a number of very active programs researching the role of diet, supplements and nutrition in prostate cancer. The U.S. government, through the National Cancer Institute and the National Institutes of Health, is providing increased funding for research into the role of diet and nutrition in cancer prevention and cancer treatment.

What can I do to reduce my risks of getting or dying of prostate cancer?
Anything that is good for your heart or promotes longevity is good for your prostate health. If it is heart healthy, it is prostate healthy. The goal is a longevity lifestyle to include commonsense suggestions for a high-variety, well-balanced diet, limiting total caloric intake to what you need, keeping your cholesterol in check, avoiding obesity, exercising regularly, eliminating tobacco and restricting alcohol intake. Interestingly, the larger your waist, the higher your risks for cancer and other diseases.

Does diet play a role in prostate cancer?
Yes. Studies suggest that a high-fat diet stimulates prostate cancer to grow. This is particularly true of red meat and dairy products. Prostate cancer is far less common in countries with a low-fat diet, such as Japan and China. When men from those countries move to countries with high-fat diets, the risks of developing prostate cancer increase and may be as high as everyone else's within a generation or two. This suggests that diet is probably one of the factors that enables or perhaps even encourages the cancers to grow. Cancer growth can be influenced at many stages of growth by nutrition.

How does a high-fat diet stimulate prostate cancer?
It probably serves to activate an otherwise dormant internal mechanism within a cell's own structure that directs the cell to grow without its usual limits and boundaries. Or it may block a protective mechanism, so the cell can grow without its usual restrictions. Another theory suggests that excess fat that cannot be broken down into cholesterol stimulates the growth of testosterone and testosterone-like hormones, which further stimulates prostate cancer to grow. I recently spoke with an expert on livestock nutrition, and he had concerns that the pesticides and toxins a cow is exposed to and eats over its lifetime are concentrated in the fat, which we then eat and store in our bodies.

Is there anything I can eat that will reduce my chances of cancer?

Yes. Studies show that a low-fat diet high in fresh herbs and colorful fruits and vegetables—the more colorful, the better—can reduce one's risk of developing cancer because those vegetables contain more beneficial nutrients. The less-cooked these vegetables are, the higher the nutrient level. Try to eat a wide variety of healthy foods, and try to keep less than 20% of your calories from fat.

?

Can I just take supplements rather than eat the food itself?

The natural source of the nutrients is always the best source of the beneficial vitamins, minerals and antioxidants. It is always smarter to seek out fresh fruits and vegetables rather than rely on store-bought supplements. Remember, they are called "supplements," not "replacements." If you use them, use them to supplement an intelligent and balanced diet. Many experts feel that the benefits from a healthy diet cannot be replaced by simply taking some vitamins and supplements.

What should I eat more of to prevent prostate cancer?
Specifically, you should increase your intake of soy (tofu and soy milk), tomatoes (especially tomato juice, sauce and paste), green tea, red grapes (yes, including red wine or red grape juice), strawberries, raspberries, blueberries, peas, watermelon, rosemary, garlic and citrus. Use extra-virgin olive oil. Omega-3 fatty acids from fish have been shown to be beneficial. Flaxseed is fine, though ocean sources of omega-3 fatty acids are better. It is best to avoid flaxseed oil as the source of your omega-3 fatty acids.

Do the supplements always contain what they claim?
Sadly, no. What is in each capsule can vary widely from capsule to capsule within the same bottle and from jar to jar. And even if the supplement is there, it may not be in a form useable by the body.

If taking recommended doses is good for me, will taking a lot more be even more beneficial?
Absolutely not. In fact, some megadoses of vitamins and supplements are actually quite dangerous and are known to increase your risks for some cancers. We know that huge megadoses may actually be worse for cancer prevention and treatment.

I had thought David M., a businessman in his early 60s with a fairly aggressive prostate cancer, understood the importance of diet and nutrition. After a successful prostatectomy, he returned for his follow-up visit. I learned that he continued to eat a high-fat diet. He felt that as long as he took a few supplements, he was fine. He didn't understand that supplements alone weren't going to make a difference—until the cancer returned. Then he agreed to change his diet. Following additional treatments and a change in his diet, David is doing well, with no evidence of cancer recurrence.

What are antioxidants?

Though oxygen is essential to life, after its use in the cells, high-energy toxic molecules are formed. Called "free radicals," or *oxidants*, these high-energy particles actually damage normal cells. In fact, many experts believe that most cancers and even aging itself are a result of the buildup of this oxidative damage over a lifetime. *Antioxidants* are chemicals the body uses to neutralize the potentially damaging effects of oxidants.

Does taking vitamin supplements work as well as eating vegetables?

No, not at all. Currently it is suggested that you get the nutrients you need from fresh fruits and vegetables. No definite research studies show that taking vitamins in pill or liquid form provides the same benefits we see with eating fresh fruits and vegetables. In fact, recent studies suggest that taking regular vitamins or supplements may not offer any advantage. Again, seek out the natural food source for these nutrients.

How can I increase the level of antioxidants in my body?

The best way is through a diet that is high in herbs, fruits and vegetables that contain large amounts of the necessary micronutrients and antioxidants that your body needs to eliminate the dangerous oxidants. In fact, the bright colors of fruits and vegetables are a way of identifying those high in antioxidants.

> *Common sense should always apply. These dietary points are guidelines—not strict rules.*

What foods should I avoid?
Red meat (beef, pork and lamb) and high-fat dairy products have been directly linked as stimulators of prostate cancer and should be avoided. Any food in moderation is fine. Excess fat intake from meat or dairy should be avoided.

What if I am served beef at a friend's house? Will one meal hurt me?
Common sense should always apply. These dietary points are guidelines for an intelligent diet—they are not strict rules. Moderation is the key.

Is it true that an Italian diet is considered healthful?
Ideally, the goal should be a Southern Mediterranean diet—one high in garlic, tomatoes, red wine and fresh fruits and vegetables, low in beef and dairy products. In addition, a rural-Japanese diet is considered healthful—high in fresh vegetables, minimal meat, plenty of soy and green tea.

Will it do me any good to eat differently now that I have prostate cancer?
Most likely. It is always a good idea to eat a balanced diet with a variety of healthful foods and avoid foods shown to have harmful effects. It is believed that a healthful low-fat diet may reduce the odds of developing cancer or could even slow down a cancer you already have.

DESIRABLE FRESH FOODS

Herbs	Watermelon	Red grapes	Blueberries
Peas	Broccoli	(including red	Fish
Apples	Tomatoes	wine or red	Green tea
Spinach	Raspberries	grape juice)	
Soy	Rosemary	Strawberries	
Citrus	Cauliflower	Aged garlic	

> *Why are tomatoes and many red vegetables and fruits so healthful?*
>
> ?
>
> Lycopene is a natural substance that gives tomatoes and other vegetables their red color. It is a very powerful anticancer chemical that may reduce the risk of cancer. Lycopene has been shown to prevent and slow the growth of cancer cells in the lab. As you increase your intake of these anticancer nutrients, you may reduce your chances of developing prostate cancer. In the future, this new area of research may provide medications to treat or prevent prostate cancer. Foods that are high in lycopene include tomatoes and tomato products (such as ketchup, tomato sauce, tomato paste), watermelon, papaya, guava, apricots and pink grapefruit.

I've heard about beta-carotene. Is this helpful with prostate cancer?

Beta-carotene is a vitamin found in leafy green vegetables and carrots. It looks very good as a beneficial dietary ingredient to reduce cancer growth. Variations of beta-carotene are even being used as a formal treatment for some types of cancer. Beta-carotene may have a protective mechanism that works to slow down the rapid cell growth that is seen with cancers. Whether it will be of use with prostate cancer is not yet proven.

What foods are high in beta-carotene?

Foods high in beta-carotene include dark-green, leafy vegetables, broccoli, spinach, romaine lettuce, beets, Swiss chard, kale, carrots, tomatoes, sweet potatoes and yams. Many cruciferous vegetables decrease risks for developing prostate and other cancers.

What are the benefits of taking vitamin E?

Some studies show that supplementing your diet with vitamin E may have some benefit in preventing and treating prostate cancer. Vitamin E is thought to boost the body's immune system and fight free radicals, and it may decrease the death rate from prostate cancer. A recent study though showed no benefit from vitamin E in preventing prostate cancer, so the answer is

Does taking a selenium supplement reduce my risk of developing prostate cancer?

Yes, for men who have low selenium levels, taking a daily selenium supplement may reduce risks of cancer and may even slow down cancer that is already present. The same study that showed no benefit in taking vitamin E also showed no benefit in taking selenium. If your selenium intake is good and you have normal levels from food sources, taking selenium won't help. Good sources of selenium include Brazil nuts (not shelled), fish, shellfish, whole grain foods, poultry and lean meats, mushrooms, eggs, onions and garlic.

still out. I prefer the natural vitamin E (d-alpha), which is much better absorbed than the synthetic (dl-alpha). Again, eating foods high in vitamin E is the best way to ingest these nutrients. Sources of natural vitamin E include vegetables, healthy vegetable oils (olive oil, canola, and soybean oil), nuts (almonds), sunflower seeds and egg yolks.

Can taking vitamin E be dangerous for some people?
Yes. Men who have bleeding problems or who take blood thinners must get approval from their doctors before taking any vitamin E, because the interaction of their drug and vitamin E can be dangerous. You should stop taking vitamin E several weeks before any surgery or biopsy.

Why is selenium important in our diet?
Selenium is a trace mineral that serves as one of the key elements of our body's antioxidant immune system. Selenium was originally obtained from the soil after flooding. Artificial fertilizers and controlled waterways have dramatically reduced the selenium that is available to our crops. Certain areas in the United States and the world are naturally low in this mineral, and those who live there often have low selenium levels and higher rates of many cancers. Selenium is found in seafood, meats and Brazil nuts. Selenium is inexpensive, easy to mass-produce and relatively safe even at high doses. The

exact dose that is most beneficial and safe has yet to be determined. For now, if you are not involved in a research study, 200 micrograms daily seems to be a safe dose. Selenium has been reported to detoxify environmental poisons and toxins in our bodies, boost the immune system and strengthen the heart, as well as prevent and possibly treat some cancers. Selenium is an essential supplement for livestock around the world.

What is good about soy?

Soy contains a number of very powerful plant substances called *phytoestrogens*, which are naturally occurring substances that resemble estrogen. In dietary doses, they can reduce risks for prostate cancer. Some believe that the active ingredients of soy actually block angiogenesis. Some doctors are even prescribing soy in larger doses to help control cancer growth once it has been detected. Good sources are soybeans, tofu, and miso soup.

How are green tea and red grapes helpful?

Green tea has been found to contain very powerful antioxidants that help to stabilize the cells and reduce damage that can progress to cancer. Some experts recommend four to five cups a day or the equivalent in capsules. Red grapes and red wines are also high in different but equally powerful antioxidants. Eating red grapes daily is suggested, as well as drinking red grape juice or red wine each day (no, not the entire bottle!). Many of their substances block cancer cell growth.

Do pesticides and chemicals play a role in prostate cancer?

Though there is no proof, some scientists are concerned that the excess chemicals we eat daily on our fruits and vegetables and in meat may be accumulating in our bodies and possibly triggering or stimulating cancer growth. Eating organic foods may help to reduce this problem, as well as washing all fruits and vegetables that you and your family eat. Dr. Frank Whiting, a cattle nutritionist, worries about the harmful toxins that accumulate in the animal fat we eat. Pesticides and other chemicals used on the feed are eaten by the cow and then stored in the muscle fat. The fear is that when you eat meat from this cow, you are getting the combined lifetime of chemicals that accumulated in that cow. Perhaps it is not the fat but these pesticides and toxins that are stimulating cancer growth.

Why can't we reduce the risks of prostate cancer with diet alone?
An individual can lower his risk of prostate cancer by following correct, life-long dietary practices. However, our industrialized Western population is not likely to change to a high-fiber, low-fat diet. Therefore, it is highly unlikely that the incidence of prostate cancer will ever be reduced by dietary changes alone.

What about herbs?
Recent studies show that the highest levels of antioxidants are found in *fresh* herbs, such as oregano, peppermint, rosemary and thyme.

Does it make a difference how much I eat?
Yes, researchers have demonstrated that a high calorie intake is not healthy. Longevity is associated with a low-calorie diet. You should eat enough at a meal to last until the next meal. Instead, too many people eat as if it will be the last meal they eat for weeks. Again, intelligent moderation is the key. Enjoy the meal, but don't go back for seconds and thirds.

I have heard so much about fish oil. Is this good to take?
The nutrients from fish oil, the omega-3 fatty acids, are essential for normal prostate and heart health. The best sources are cold-water fish, such as salmon, cod, herring, mackerel, sardines, tuna, and anchovies (yes, an-chovies). Another source is fresh flaxseed, but the fish source is better. You should avoid flaxseed oil because it deteriorates quickly, becoming rancid. In addition, flaxseed oil creates a variety of less desirable acids in addition to the healthy omega-3 fatty acids.

What else can I do to reduce my risks for prostate cancer?
In addition to eating a smart diet with a lot of variety, being sure to get plenty of fiber can help reduce your risks for a number of problems and cancers.

Why is a high calcium intake bad for prostate cancer?
When you take a high dose of calcium, you block your body's production of its own internal form of vitamin D, which is thought to block cancer cell growth. Some men with low vitamin D levels have higher rates of cancer. If your levels are low, your doctor may ask to start vitamin D supplements. The best source of vitamin D is daily sunshine, in moderation of course. Interestingly, men with skin cancer from too much sun have lower rates of prostate cancer.

Is it true that anticholesterol medications may help?
Yes, research suggests that taking statins to lower your cholesterol may reduce your risk for getting prostate cancer.

Are there reliable sources on nutrition and cancer?
For more information on diet and prostate cancer, Dr. Charles Myers at the University of Virginia publishes a monthly newsletter about prostate cancer and nutrition. The newsletter is called the *Prostate Forum,* and it is an excellent resource, and the only one specifically about prostate cancer prevention and treatment. I subscribe. For more information, call 1-800-305-2432. I also receive the *Tufts University Health & Nutrition Letter,* which is considered an excellent resource on all aspects of nutrition and health. To order, call 1-800-274-7581.

SYMPTOMS OF CANCER

4

Prostate cancer progresses from a point at which the tumor is small and has no effect on surrounding tissues and organs, to such a size that it affects the body in a number of different ways. A man usually seeks medical attention when he first becomes aware that something isn't right.

When you have an appointment with your doctor, you will be asked about your past medical problems, past surgery, medications you take (including the specific names, dosages, and how often they are taken) and any allergies you may know about. You should also provide the names and doses of *all* supplements, herbs, vitamins and minerals you take.

You will also be asked about the history of serious illnesses or health problems in your family, whether you smoke or drink alcohol and how much. The doctor will want to know about any problems you may be experiencing that may serve as clues regarding underlying disorders. These are called *symptoms*.

Symptoms of Concern

What are the warning symptoms that I might have prostate cancer?
Unfortunately, there are *no* early warnings that prostate cancer may be growing in your body. In fact, most often there are no warning signs or symptoms at all.

Prostate cancer usually grows very slowly. Because of its location in the prostate, it usually doesn't cause physical symptoms. Even when it causes symptoms, they are not specific, meaning that those symptoms could represent a number of problems other than prostate cancer. The same nonspecific symptoms of prostate enlargement could also be caused by an enlarging prostate cancer as it compresses the urethra.

Could I have prostate cancer and have no symptoms?
It is quite possible. This does occur, far too often, with men being diagnosed with large and advanced cancers even though they deny having urination problems. We are diagnosing more men with absolutely no symptoms even when the cancer may be significant and potentially life threatening.

Are there any ways to know that I have prostate cancer if there are no symptoms early on?
The best way to detect prostate cancer early is by a physical exam of the prostate and the PSA blood test. Each of these alone is helpful. But together, if you have a potentially dangerous cancer, the exam and PSA are likely to

How can I have cancer if I feel so good and have no symptoms?

This is a common discussion between urologists and their patients who have just been diagnosed with prostate cancer. This illustrates the point I am trying to make: There are *no* early warning signs. If you wait until something is obviously wrong, then most likely you have waited too long. The disease could be in an advanced stage. This is why a routine annual exam by your physician should always include a prostate check and a PSA blood test.

indicate abnormalities. Prostate cancer, if it grows large enough, will lead to the onset of exactly the same bothersome symptoms as a noncancerous prostate growth.

What are the symptoms of an enlarged prostate that might disguise a growing prostate cancer?

Some prostate-enlargement symptoms include:

- Getting up at night to urinate.
- Urinating frequently during the daytime.
- Standing a long time before the urinary stream starts.
- Lots of dribbling at the end of the stream.
- A sense of urgency to rush to the bathroom.
- Leakage of urine.
- Straining to empty your bladder.
- Returning to the bathroom to urinate again just a few minutes after completion of urinating

If I have prostate cancer, will I have all of these symptoms?

Most likely, no. You may have any combination of symptoms—just a few, all of them or none at all.

Are there any symptoms if the cancer has spread?

This depends on where the cancer has spread. Back, rib, hip or shoulder pain could suggest that prostate cancer has spread to the bones. Often the pains will come and go. Fatigue, weakness, or generalized aches and pains could also represent prostate cancer in more advanced stages. Rarely, advanced prostate cancer can cause pelvic pain or even paralysis.

All of these problems are nonspecific. In other words, they don't indicate *why* you have these symptoms. Even if there is advanced prostate cancer, most men will describe only a few symptoms at any given time. Some of these aches and pains may also just be the result of a naturally aging body. This is why a routine exam is so important. Without exception, the prostate exam should always be a part of your routine annual physical.

Roberto just couldn't believe he could have prostate cancer and not feel pain or have any symptoms. No matter how often I tried to explain it, he just couldn't accept that he had cancer. In family and friends, he had seen other cancers associated with pain or bleeding. After about six months, and multiple conversations with family members and my office, he finally agreed to proceed with radiation. He had no problems, continues to feel great, and is doing well . . . though I suspect, deep down, he still doesn't think he had prostate cancer.

Does blood in the urine suggest prostate cancer?

Most often when blood is seen in the urine (a condition called *hematuria*), it is not associated with prostate cancer. The blood may come from non-cancerous enlargement of the prostate, broken blood vessels on the surface of the prostate, prostate or bladder infections, bladder tumors or even kidney stones or tumors. Sometimes, we never find the source.

Is it possible to have blood in the urine if you have cancer?

Yes, it is possible. Because the presence of blood may be an indication of something serious, it is very important to have a complete urologic evaluation when you have bloody urine, even just one time.

Should I worry if I see blood in my semen?

Usually not. Most often blood in the semen, called *hematospermia*, is not associated with prostate cancer. Rather, it is thought to come from inflammation or irritation of the prostate or seminal vesicles. This inflamation or irritation may be seen with an infection, following straining during sexual

CAUSES OF BLOOD IN THE URINE

Enlarged prostate	Bladder infection
Bladder stones	Kidney cancer
Prostate cancer	Bladder cancer
Kidney stones	Unknown source

activity or after a bowel movement. The majority of times the evaluation is completely normal, and there is no evidence of cancer in the prostate.

However, nothing is 100% sure, so it is always possible that blood in the semen may be a warning sign of something wrong with the prostate, such as cancer. It is always important to see a urologist regarding blood in the semen to be certain everything is normal. Don't just assume that nothing is wrong. The evaluation is quick, and the knowledge that there is no cancer is reassuring.

THE DIGITAL RECTAL EXAM (DRE)

5

Because of the prostate gland's location, one major aspect of your physical exam is most important—the digital rectal exam (DRE). This three- to four-second procedure can detect abnormalities years before symptoms develop. The exam should be a regular part of your annual visit to the doctor.

What is the purpose of the physical exam?
The doctor wants to make sure there are no abnormal changes or irregularities indicating that something could be wrong. Your urine is checked for abnormalities (it should be clear usually), and blood will be drawn from a vein for analysis. Anything wrong that the doctor can see, feel or detect is called a *sign*.

Every man over the age of 50 should routinely have a general medical exam, a digital rectal exam, a urine evaluation and a PSA blood test. These can be done at the same time when you visit your primary-care doctor. The information provided by all of these functions can help your physician decide if there is reason to be concerned. If something is not as it should be, then further evaluation may be appropriate.

One of my favorite patients, Craig, was told by his primary doctor that he had a nodule on his prostate. This doctor said they could monitor the situation, and if it changed over several years, he'd refer Craig to a urologist. After doing some reading, Craig called me and made an appointment for evaluation on his own. Sure enough, it was a very suspicious lump. Further testing confirmed it was a fairly significant cancer, and Craig underwent successful surgery. Craig had a large cancer, close to spreading outside of the gland. Only after the surgery did Craig tell me his primary doctor had wanted him to watch the lump grow over several years. By that time, it would most certainly have spread.

What exactly is a prostate exam?

The exam is primarily a feel of the back wall of the prostate gland. This exam goes by a variety of different names, including *rectal exam, DRE, digital exam, prostate exam* and *finger wave*. I had one patient who wondered how I could do a digital exam without a computer. He thought *digital* meant *computer* and did not realize the finger is referred to as a *digit*.

To do the exam, your doctor briefly inserts a gloved, lubricated finger into the rectum to feel the back wall of the prostate gland. Some rectal cancers can be felt, providing additional potentially lifesaving information.

Does the exam let the doctor feel the entire gland?

No. The exam allows for feeling only the back wall of the gland. This is like feeling the back of your head and trying to guess what your face looks like. Much of the prostate cannot be felt during the rectal exam.

What is the doctor trying to feel?

The doctor will feel for any areas of firmness or hard nodules, lumps or irregularities. I am basically feeling to see if there are any areas that are not soft, smooth and symmetrical. If something is not right, it simply suggests that cancer *may* be present. An abnormality does *not* always mean cancer! A number of other things can cause abnormalities in the exam. These include

> *If there is an irregularity, should I just wait and see if it changes over time?*
>
> No, this is not a wise choice. This approach was popular many years ago and still leads to unnecessary problems today. Even if the PSA test is normal, an irregularity in the prostate gland could possibly represent a serious but *curable* cancer. If you were to leave and return for a repeat exam six months later and the irregularity were even bigger, then you may have lost that opportunity to detect and treat the cancer while it was still confined to the prostate gland.

previous surgery of the prostate, past or present prostate infections, prior biopsies, stones in the prostate and even noncancerous growths that can cause nodules.

Should I have my annual exam done by a urologist?

Not usually. This decision depends on how skilled and experienced your primary-care doctor is at performing and interpreting the exam. In my practice, most of the abnormalities picked up on the exam are felt by the primary-care doctors. They then send the patient to me for a consultation.

I still see a number of men, however, who prefer to have a urologist perform their annual exam. There is some truth to the old statement that checking prostates is what urologists do for a living. All things being equal, if the primary-care doctor doesn't feel an irregularity or nodule, it is not common for me to detect something. Occasionally I do, but not often.

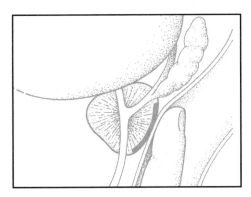

PROSTATE EXAMINATION. Digital rectal examination allows the examiner's finger to feel only the back wall of the prostate, adjacent to the rectal wall. Cancers in the middle or front of the prostate might not be felt.

Does it matter if I see different doctors for my exam each year?
Yes. Ideally, you should have your exam done by the same person each year so that, if there are any subtle changes, your doctor will be able to detect them. If at all possible, try to find a doctor you have confidence in and have that doctor do your examination every year.

What if my doctor does my regular examination and does not do a rectal exam?
You should insist on one. Your doctor can detect a prostate or even rectal cancer early only if he or she does the exam. When a doctor does not do a rectal exam on a male patient it makes me a little uncomfortable. Why wouldn't a doctor do it? It is, after all, a very important part of every exam.

Does taking Avodart or Proscar impact on my exam?
Interestingly, if you take one of these prostate-shrinking medications, the doctor will be able to better detect a cancer than on men not on those medications. This is thought to occur because it is easier to feel a hard lump of cancer if the prostate is smaller.

PSA BLOOD TEST— KEY DETECTION TOOL

6

Prostate specific antigen (PSA) is the single most valuable tumor marker available. The PSA blood test has revolutionized the detection of prostate cancer. Without a doubt, this single test accounts for early detection and cure of prostate cancer in many tens of thousands of individuals each year. The use of PSA testing has led to a dramatic reduction in men diagnosed with advanced prostate cancer.

Though far from perfect, the PSA blood test and the digital rectal exam, when used together correctly, provide the best information needed to tell if a cancer may be present in the prostate gland. We know the PSA test significantly increases our ability to detect cancers early, years before they can be felt on the exam.

What is PSA?

PSA stands for *prostate specific antigen.* It is an enzyme in the blood that is normally produced by prostate cells, both normal and cancerous. PSA is found nowhere else in the body in significant amounts. Normally, a small amount of PSA is constantly released into the bloodstream. When the prostate is irritated, is damaged or turns cancerous, more of the PSA leaks out and can be measured by the PSA blood test. This is why the PSA test is very sensitive to identifying any abnormalities of the prostate, including but not limited to prostate cancer.

A mild to moderate increase in PSA does *not* mean you definitely have cancer. PSA is prostate specific, not cancer specific. A change in the level suggests there is an increased *possibility* of having cancer. Many times no cancer is detected. However, a very high PSA level is very suggestive of a cancer because one of the characteristics of cancer cells is that they release ten times more PSA into the bloodstream than normal prostate cells.

What is the normal range for the PSA levels?

The normal range is between 0.0 and 2.5. The old cutoff of 4.0 failed to detect a significant number of men with prostate cancer, and so was abandoned. Studies have revealed that the trend of the PSA over time (PSA velocity) is even more important at picking up potentially life-threatening prostate cancers early. The PSA when considered in relation to the prostate size is also important (PSA density). Of concern is an elevated PSA with a small prostate size.

How quickly can I get several PSA levels to check my PSA velocity?

You will need at least two, and ideally three, routine PSA results spread out over two years. Because of normal fluctuations in the testing, checking levels more often doesn't help and actually may be confusing.

Does my age have anything to do with the PSA?

Many experts believe in using the "age-related" PSA exam. We know that the PSA level normally increases as men age. Dr. William Catalona and his

AGE-RELATED PSA

Age	Max level	African American men
40–50	2.5	2.0
50–60	3.5	3.0
65 and older	4.0	4.0

colleagues determined that younger men should have lower PSA levels than older men.

Studies by Judd Moul, M.D., of Duke University show that the upper limit of normal for African American men should be even lower to detect cancer early while it may still be curable. In black men between the ages of 40 and 49, the upper limit of PSA should be 2.0.

How high does the PSA go?

Though most men with prostate cancer are diagnosed with a PSA level from 3 to 15, the PSA can go into the hundreds and even the thousands. A reading at these higher levels almost always means you have advanced prostate cancer. Often additional tests will show the cancer may have spread to the bones or the lymph nodes. I have seen some men with prostate infections that push the PSA reading up over 100 or higher, but with treatment it returns to normal within a few months.

What can cause an increase in the PSA level?

The PSA can be elevated for a number of reasons. Anything that irritates the prostate can push up the PSA level. Irritations include any inflammation or infection of the prostate, simple enlargement or noncancerous growth of the prostate gland (there is more tissue to produce PSA), prostate cancer, stones within the prostate, a recent urinary catheter or procedure, recent prostate biopsies or prostate or bladder surgery.

What is the "free-to-total" and "complexed PSA"?

A new aspect of the PSA test looks at components of PSA in the bloodstream to determine how much PSA is bound (complexed) to proteins and how much is free (unbound). This is then calculated as the free PSA–to–total PSA ratio. The *higher* the number, the less likely cancer is the cause of the total PSA elevation.

Like the free-to-total PSA, a complexed PSA is another variant that helps raise or lower our level of suspicion about the presence of cancer. The free form of PSA (not complexed) is seen more in men without prostate cancer. I have found the free-to-total and complexed PSA to be very helpful in detecting significant cancer even when the PSA is considered normal.

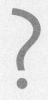

Can infections elsewhere in the body cause an elevation of the PSA?

Infections elsewhere in the body cannot elevate the PSA level. Colds, flu, pneumonia and all other nonurinary infections will not elevate the PSA result.

Does a urinary-tract infection elevate the PSA level very much?

Yes, the PSA level can rise substantially because of inflammation in the prostate gland from the infection. I have seen the PSA level go as high as 120 and then drop back down to 2.5 eight weeks after an infection was treated. It is important to allow enough time for the irritation to resolve.

How long after a urinary-tract or prostate infection should I wait to have a PSA test?

First, the infection has to be adequately treated with the correct antibiotics. A urine culture is usually obtained to identify the infection. Then we can see which antibiotics will work. You should be on antibiotics for two to four weeks.

Even after the infection is over, there still is residual inflammation and irritation that needs to resolve before the PSA will drop to your normal level. The PSA should normally be checked eight weeks or more after the infection is over. I also often do a follow-up urine test about a week or two after the antibiotic treatment to be sure the infection is totally gone.

I'm really afraid my high PSA isn't because of my infection. Will waiting for it to go down hurt me?

No. There are no guarantees, but most patients who had a high PSA level as well as a urinary-tract infection had a normal PSA level after the infection was treated and the inflammation subsided.

My PSA level jumped dramatically. Does that mean I have a bad cancer?

Probably not. In fact, a dramatic jump in PSA is almost always from infection or other noncancerous causes. Cancer does push the PSA up, but not usually that fast.

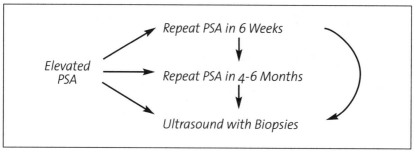

Options for elevated PSA with normal digital exam of the prostate.

Why do you have to wait so long to recheck the PSA?

I am asked this all the time. It takes a long time for the swelling and irritation of the tissues of the prostate gland to heal. If the PSA is checked while the swelling and irritation are still present, then the PSA level will still be elevated and will continue to confuse the issue. You should wait long enough for healing before the PSA test is performed again.

If the PSA test doesn't confirm cancer, why do it?

I prefer to consider an elevated PSA as a *warning sign* that cancer may be present, then do further evaluation. I often use the analogy that the PSA test is like a red warning light in your car's dashboard. It tells you something may be wrong, but it doesn't tell you what. The higher the PSA level, the more likely a cancer is present and the more likely cancer will be a threat to your life. Even mild elevations can suggest a cancer is present. The key is to find the cancer when it is still small, confined to the prostate and easily treatable.

CAUSES OF ELEVATED PSA

- Cancer of prostate
- Urinary-tract infection
- Prostatitis (prostate infection)
- Stones within prostate
- Catheter in bladder/urinary retention
- Recent prostate surgery
  - Laser
  - TURP
- Recent prostate biopsies
- Noncancerous enlargement of prostate gland

?

If my PSA level is normal, does that mean I don't have cancer?

A normal PSA level does not mean you don't have cancer. It simply means you are less likely to have cancer. I have had patients with a PSA level as low as 0.9 who had a significant cancer. The PSA test is just one investigative tool.

If the PSA level is elevated, is the digital prostate exam always abnormal?

No, not usually. If the PSA level is up, the digital exam is often normal. Conversely, if you have an abnormal digital exam from an aggressive cancer, the PSA may or may not be elevated. Most often you will be told you have an elevated PSA level, even though your digital exam is normal. The PSA level simply serves as a warning test and gives us an early clue before the digital exam shows any change. We use the PSA test as a measure of probability.

Why would the digital exam be "normal" if the PSA is high?

If the cancer is not along the back wall where we feel with an exam, and instead is located in the middle or even the front of the prostate, then the digital exam often won't detect the abnormality.

At what PSA level should I be concerned?

If your digital exam is normal and the PSA level is well within the normal range, you can probably feel comfortable. Everything is probably fine. The PSA should stay at about the same level every time it is checked. There may be a slight increase over time as you age and your prostate gradually enlarges. There will also be some minor fluctuations and variability.

As an example, one of my patients was very upset that his PSA level went from 1.5 to 1.7 over a six-month period. I explained that this probably represents the usual day-to-day fluctuations in the level.

The point is, look at the general range and do not focus on the specific number. Is the PSA low, mildly elevated or high? Don't overemphasize the particular number. The trend of your PSA levels over years (PSA velocity) is felt by many to be more important than the numbers themselves.

When should I have the PSA test done?

Most men have the PSA test every year, starting no later than at age 50. I suggest a baseline level at ages 40 and 45 to have for reference before you get older. Getting tested once a year after age 50 is adequate. More often doesn't seem to help, and less often may let some cancers grow too long before being detected. If you are in a high-risk group, meaning more likely to have cancer, then you should start your annual checks at age 40. This applies to men with a family history of prostate cancer (father, brother, uncle, grandfather) and African American men.

My PSA level has always been very low but just went up, though it is still normal. Should I be concerned?

An unexpected change in the PSA number is always of concern and warrants a complete evaluation, no matter what the number is.

Recently, I was following the progress of a man with a normal exam and a PSA around 1.0 every year for several years. A follow-up exam was still normal, but his PSA jumped up to 2.6. I checked, and he had no infection or reason to explain the sudden elevation. Subsequent evaluation showed he did have cancer of the prostate. He opted for surgery, which showed a surprisingly large volume of cancer but no evidence the cancer had spread. He has an excellent long-term prognosis.

What is the value of checking PSA levels for men in their 40s?

The ideal average PSA for men in their 40s is a level between 0.6 and 0.7. If the PSA is higher than this age-specific level, it raises concerns that something could be starting, so annual checks and close monitoring are important.

What does the PSA blood test cost?

The test itself should cost between $40 and $85, depending on your location. It is almost always covered by your insurance plan or Medicare.

Almost all insurance plans realize there is a benefit to early detection and treatment of prostate cancer. The test is so important that I strongly suggest you pay for it yourself if that's what is necessary to get it done. You may be able to find a prostate-screening program that offers the test for around $15 to $20.

What if my doctor doesn't want to do a PSA test?

This happens occasionally. Many primary-care doctors have become confused by arguments about whether doctors are changing anything with early detection and treatment. I believe the facts today support early detection of a potentially lethal cancer.

Your primary-care doctor may say he or she does not think a PSA test is needed. You can explain that you have done your own research, and although you realize it is not proven 100 percent, the majority of prostate cancer experts still do recommend a PSA test. You can emphasize that you feel very strongly about having the test.

Why is there so much confusion and controversy about the use of PSA testing to detect prostate cancer by primary-care doctors?

Unfortunately, many leading organizations have come out and formally announced that before a PSA test is performed, you should be counseled by your primary-care doctor on all of the following: the pros and cons of PSA testing, other possible tests that may be required if questions are raised by the PSA, the pros and cons of those associated tests, and the pros and cons of prostate-cancer treatment options.

It is not likely that most primary-care physicians can take 20 minutes to explain all this to you. And to ask them to do so isn't very realistic. My personal belief is that you have chosen your particular doctor because you trust him or her to take the best care of you and to do whatever it takes to keep you healthy throughout your life. When your doctor wants to do a chest X-ray and EKG, or check your blood for cholesterol, he or she doesn't take 30 minutes to counsel you on the potential risks or pros and cons of the lab tests. Does your doctor spend 30 minutes talking with your wife about the pros and cons of ordering a mammogram? Unlikely. The doctor orders the test because it is felt to be a helpful tool in providing state-of-the-art care. It is all about keeping you alive and healthy. In a like manner, I believe that the PSA exam is an important test that should be done routinely. What we do

Retired engineers and scientists are some of my best patients, but sometimes they have a hard time with the art, in contrast to the science, of medicine. My patient Tom was one such person. He kept a detailed computerized record of his PSA tests following treatment for his cancer. It was hard for Tom to accept that a test couldn't be perfect and consistent each and every time. One day he called, very upset because his PSA level had jumped from 0.4 to 0.6, an increase of 50%. I explained the variability of the test to him again. I asked him not to worry and to repeat the test. Sure enough, the next text came back at 0.3 and Tom relaxed—until the next normal fluctuation.

with the results requires some knowledge of what the PSA is and what it isn't, and a little common sense.

Is there an age when I should not get the PSA test?

Yes. The basic guideline I use is this: If you will not allow the doctor to do anything if a cancer is found—because either you think you are too sick or too old—then there really is no reason to undergo the blood test and any additional evaluation. Why take the risks of a biopsy and endure the anxiety if it's not going to make a difference?

At some point in your life, you should sit back and realize that even if you have some prostate cancer, it probably will not cause any problems or shorten your life span. That is the point at which to stop checking a PSA.

As we were taught in medical school, don't take the temperature if you don't want to find a fever. I suggest men stop checking their PSA levels when they feel they are too old to benefit from the information, or if they will not allow any treatments. Men who are still healthy, active and vibrant may want to continue checking their PSA level, especially if they have longevity in their family. The general guideline is to stop checking the PSA level if you have a normal exam and less than a ten-year life expectancy. One way of looking at it is to say if you are older than 75 or 80, you should stop checking your PSA unless you have significant longevity in the family, with one or both parents living into their late 80s or 90s.

Will my doctor call and remind me to get my PSA done?
Probably not. A doctor's office with thousands of patients can't be expected to remind each one of routine lab tests.

Take control of your own health and put it on your schedule. Don't assume you don't need a PSA recheck just because your doctor didn't call and tell you so. I have seen patients who have disappeared, only to return a few years later with extensive cancer because they assumed their doctor would track them down to remind them about their annual PSA and exam.

Does it make a difference if I have the test before or after the digital prostate exam?
We used to think so, but studies show it doesn't make a difference. If your doctor did not do a vigorous prostate massage, you can have the PSA test done right after the exam. In general, most men can have a PSA blood sample drawn after a routine prostate exam without concern that it may push up the level.

Does the PSA test tell whether or not I should have surgery?
No, but if you have cancer, the PSA test can be a useful tool to help doctors decide whether the cancer is confined to the prostate. If the PSA level is less than 4.0, it is likely the cancer will be confined to the prostate. If the PSA level is greater than 10.0, it is more likely the cancer will have started to grow through the wall and possibly outside the prostate's capsule and into surrounding fat or even into the seminal vesicles.

Does the PSA level reveal anything about the cancer if it is present?
The higher the PSA, the larger the cancer tends to be. The larger the cancer, the more aggressive the cancer cells are.

For reasons I can't explain, someone's PSA score may occasionally be inaccurately high. When in doubt, check it again. If it remains elevated, then you should seek evaluation by a urologist.

*If I have an elevated PSA level with an abnormal digital exam, should
I also get a recheck of the PSA?*

No, if there is an irregularity on the prostate, then that is reason enough to
proceed with further evaluation and biopsy, so I don't recommend a recheck.

*Does the PSA tell anything about which treatment options may be best
or should be avoided?*

To some degree, yes. As the PSA goes higher and higher, the chance increases
that the cancer has spread outside the prostate. Many urologists will recommend radiation if they don't believe that surgery will be curative. But the
PSA test alone doesn't give a definitive diagnosis. It's a lab test that helps the
doctor interpret all the information when making a diagnosis and determining treatment options. It is just a piece of the puzzle.

Can the PSA test indicate whether cancer has spread?

Only if the PSA level is very elevated, above 70 or more in most men. The
cancer could very well be in lymph nodes or in bone at much lower levels,
but you cannot assume that is true in everybody unless the PSA level is very
elevated. Again, the higher the PSA score, the more likely it is that the cancer
has spread.

*Does it make a difference if I've been fasting before blood is drawn for
the PSA test?*

No. You can have the blood drawn for the PSA test whether you have eaten
recently or not. What you eat does not influence the PSA level.

Will any medications change my PSA levels?

Early studies suggest that regularly taking aspirin or other anti-inflammation
medications such as ibuprofen might decrease the measured PSA levels.

*Is the PSA level really lower or is it just that somehow taking these
meds makes the PSA appear lower? And does this mean a lower chance
for cancer or could this somehow be making a higher level?*

These are questions that still need to be answered. For now, just be sure to
tell your doctor if you take these medications.

Are there any medications that affect the PSA level?

?

Yes. Proscar, Avodart and Propecia can drop the measured PSA by about 10% to 90%. In fact, if the PSA does not drop with these medications, then I would be concerned that cancer may be present. Other medications that reduce testosterone levels can also drop the PSA level as testosterone is needed for the prostate cells to produce PSA.

Can the PSA test be used after treatment?

This is actually the best use for the PSA test: to monitor a treatment to be sure it has worked and the cancer is not coming back. Each treatment has different expectations for what the PSA should be.

Does having sex increase the PSA level?

Yes, some studies show that there can be up to 10% elevation of the PSA. If there are questions, recheck the PSA level after abstaining from sex for several days.

Can having low testosterone impact on my PSA levels?

Yes, Men with low levels of testosterone can have an artificially low measured level of PSA.

Can I get a PSA test more often if I am really concerned?

If you are paying for the test yourself, you can have it done as often as you want. You only need to have it done about once a year. You could check it every six months if you are really concerned or at high risk. After treatment for cancer, we may need to monitor the PSA at three- or four-month intervals.

How often should I check my PSA level if it is elevated?

It depends on how suspicious your doctor is. For the average man with a mildly elevated PSA and normal exam, I will recheck the level within the next few months and if it is still elevated, even mildly, then I will proceed with an ultrasound and biopsy. If the result of the ultrasound and biopsy are normal, then I follow the PSA level initially in four to six months, again depending on the level of suspicion.

What if my doctor didn't check my PSA level in the past? Did he do something wrong?

No. There continues to be considerable debate about whether primary-care doctors should even be doing the PSA test. Because the answer wasn't clear, many excellent family practitioners and internists did not routinely check a PSA level on their patients.

Can I compare PSA results from different labs?

No. Different labs may use different manufacturer's tests. It is really best to have your PSA blood tests processed in the same lab or on the same equipment from year to year. If you are seeing the same physician or physician group, it will probably be the same lab over the years.

Does it make a difference which PSA test is done?

No. They all are good and consistent. I do think it is best to use the same lab for each of the PSA tests, whether it's for early detection or to follow the PSA levels after treatment. Your doctor is probably working with a lab he or she trusts.

Is the PSA result exact?

No, there is a definite amount of "noise" with the PSA level, which can fluctuate day-to-day and lab-to-lab. Some variability is expected.

Are the doctor's office labs as good as the big hospital labs?

In most situations, probably. The test itself is fairly easy to do, and it doesn't make a lot of difference who does it or where it is done. In larger labs, a pathologist who specializes in this work oversees testing. Big labs also are under more scrutiny and monitoring. Again, you should have the test performed at the same place each time to maintain continuity.

How long does it take to get PSA results back?

Depending on where the lab is, the time of day your blood is drawn and delays on weekends and holidays, results usually take from 15 minutes for an office PSA test to 24 to 72 hours. Some labs may do them only once or twice each week. This is always a good question to ask when you are having the test. The lab or your doctor should be able to give a fairly good idea of when results will be back.

Should I get copies of my PSA results?

Yes. I think it is a good idea to keep copies of important results of all tests you have. Just ask your doctor or the lab when your blood is being drawn. They are usually happy to provide a copy of the results to you.

Should I keep an ongoing record of my PSA test results?

Yes, this is a very smart idea. Whether it's tracking your annual PSA level or monitoring a PSA level every few months after a treatment, the record will keep you better informed and more in control. Occasionally, a patient points out a trend or concern I may not have seen. I have several patients who plot their PSA results on their computers, which makes trend lines even more dramatic. A Prostate Cancer Evaluation Log is included in the Appendix.

Are there any new tests to have in addition to the PSA?

Yes, the revolutionary PCA3 test has become an important new tool for your urologist. Here is how it works: You provide a small urine sample after prostate massage. The urine is then analyzed for genetic DNA markers that strongly suggest prostate cancer. A number is then calculated and sent to your urologist. High values suggest an increased risk for prostate cancer. Low numbers suggest a lower risk. Many urologists use the PCA3 after your first biopsies that show no cancer to see how likely it is that a cancer is present and if and when more biopsies are needed. A new test called annexin A3 looks like it will be a very effective urine marker to detect early prostate cancer, especially for men with minimally elevated PSA levels.

What tests are on the horizon?

A number of experimental tests, called biomarkers, appear to be helpful but are not commercially available for public use. They are still in experimental and trial phases. These include early prostate cancer antigens (EPCA), serum leptin levels, the human kallikrein 2 (hK2) test, and the insulin-like growth factor 1 (IGF 1) test.

Like the PSA, hK2 is secreted by prostate cells and may help identify men with prostate cancer. Early research suggests that when used in conjunction with the PSA test and the free-to-total PSA, the hK2 test may help to separate those who have cancer from those who have a noncancerous reason for their elevated PSA. HK2 may actually predict who will be diagnosed with prostate cancer up to 25 years before diagnosis.

Similar to the hK2 test, urokinase plasminogen activation (UPA), transforming growth factor (TGF) and the IGF tests promise in preliminary research studies to help with the early identification of prostate cancer and to improve the discrimination of benign from malignant prostate disease.

Does the time of year make a difference in my PSA levels?
Actually, there was a recent study that suggests that yes, your PSA levels can be higher in the summer months. More research on this is still needed before anyone can make a definitive statement on seasonality of PSA levels. Until we know more, if your PSA level is up, whatever time of year, you need evaluation!

Does obesity make a difference in PSA levels?
Yes, some studies suggest that obesity is associated with lowered measurable PSA levels. This could be from changes in hormones because of the extra fat cells in the body (fat cells are hormonally active) or perhaps the blood levels are simply diluted because of extra plasma volume. The exact relationship is still being evaluated; so for now, it should not play a role in understanding the significance of your PSA level.

Because African Americans have a greater concern over prostate cancer, does this mean that the PSA level isn't as important to them?
No. PSA levels are equally relevant for men of all races. Studies suggest that early education and use of PSA testing is the key. Therefore, the PSA test should be available for all men. Interestingly, looking at the PSA density (PSA compared to the prostate size) may be an especially sensitive test for black men for early diagnosis of prostate cancer.

SHOULD WE SCREEN
FOR CANCER?

7

Though we are still in the infancy of understanding prostate cancer and its treatments, experts have demonstrated a definite benefit to men treated early for prostate cancer. No longer do we see so many men with *advanced* disease walking into our office for the first time. This dramatic improvement can be directly credited to early detection and screening.

Prostate screening is the process of looking specifically for prostate cancer in a large number of men. The tests used are usually available widely and easily to anyone. Clinics, doctors' offices or hospitals will often advertise free screening for the public. Men are given a digital rectal exam and PSA blood test to see if there are any abnormalities that suggest prostate cancer.

Why is prostate screening so controversial?
There is some debate about the cost to society of this screening, in light of the results achieved. This is because for many of the men who are evaluated, some will need to undergo additional testing. Of these, only a small number will actually have cancer and require treatment. All of this effort and testing costs someone money.

Screening has an important role today and should be continued. I believe that it saves lives. Study after study shows the benefit of early detection and treatment of prostate cancer for those men who will benefit from treatment.

What is the difference between screening and early detection?

Screening means looking at large numbers of men for signs of prostate cancer, including many who may not be ill or even suspect a prostate abnormality. Screening is usually done through advertising to the mass population and is usually free.

When an individual goes to his physician for routine care, the doctor's examination of the prostate and drawing blood for a PSA test are referred to as *early detection*.

I believe there is still much controversy because so many confuse the screening of large groups of men with early detection for an individual. Population-based numbers are limited in helping the doctor predict an individual's situation.

Does screening make a difference?

Initially there was much debate on this question, but it now appears screening does increase the chance of finding a cancer before it has spread. The final statistics aren't in yet, but the early results of screening hundreds of thousands of men over the past several years suggest a definite advantage to finding cancers early, especially in men between 45 and 65 years old. Because of screening, there has been a shift in men being diagnosed with prostate cancer—it is rare now to see a new patient with advanced disease.

Why should I participate in prostate screening if I feel fine?

There are several reasons why screening for prostate cancer is important to you and society. First, despite what you may have heard or read, prostate cancer is a killer. Tens of thousands of men die of prostate cancer each year. This makes it the second-leading killer of men by cancer in the United States. The cancer may be slow growing in many men, but it can still be fatal and should not be ignored.

Second, prostate cancer can be present without any symptoms. Many doctors believe that the early discovery of cancer, especially in high-risk groups, results in improved long-term outcomes and better survival.

It used to be that about a third of men diagnosed with prostate cancer had advanced disease, often already spread to the bones. Now, with screening, early detection and awareness, only about 5% of all men diagnosed with prostate cancer have disease that is advanced.

Why is early detection important for prostate cancer?

First, prostate cancer does kill. Second, there is no curative treatment for advanced prostate cancer. And third, all cancers begin as small, organ-confined lesions something that is treatable and curable.

What will happen if I go for a prostate-cancer screening?

Usually prostate-cancer screening is simply a digital rectal exam. The office or clinic will often ask many questions regarding any difficulty urinating. They will also ask for your address and phone number so they can follow up with you and notify you in writing if there is a concern on the exam.

Sometimes the screeners will even do a free PSA blood test. Other places may charge you their cost to perform the blood test, about $15 to $20. The PSA test should be done as it is a much more sensitive detector of prostate cancer than a DRE.

Doctor's Note!

Raymond is a prominent attorney, who had been seeing his regular doctor and friend annually for a physical exam. I suppose because they were good friends, his doctor never felt comfortable doing a rectal exam. During prostate screening, which his doctor had told him wasn't needed, I detected a nodule, which turned out to be an aggressive prostate cancer. His treatment has worked, for now. But there remains a good chance the cancer might return ... and I'm sure Raymond will always have to wonder if he would have had a better chance if he had only had a digital rectal exam every year.

?

Is the PSA blood test a good screening test to detect prostate cancer?

I believe that it is. Over the years I have seen many men whose cancers were found as a result of an elevated PSA level during screening, even though their rectal exams were quite normal. The PSA can be a valuable tool to help identify cancers early— while they are still curable.

At screenings, what kind of physician does the exam?

At most screenings, urologists do the exams, although primary-care physicians occasionally are involved. The ability to identify cancers through digital rectal exams depends on the experience and skill of the examiner, regardless of his or her special medical training.

Can PSA be found in women?

Yes, trace and insignificant amounts of PSA can be found in certain tissues and fluids in women (breast cancer, breast tissue, breast fluid and other female tumors).

ULTRASOUND AND BIOPSY OF THE PROSTATE

8

I f anything suspicious or of concern is discovered on your prostate exam or PSA blood test, your doctor will recommend that you have a prostate ultrasound with biopsies.

According to prostate expert Dr. Ron Solomon in Newport Beach, California, this technique allows us to visualize the entire prostate gland with ultrasound waves. It provides information about the actual size of the prostate gland and whether there are suspicious areas or distortions of the gland caused by a possible cancer.

Most important, the ultrasound allows the urologist to focus the biopsies more accurately throughout the prostate and on high-risk areas that may be suspicious for cancer.

Prostate ultrasound has helped to dramatically improve the urologist's ability to detect cancer in an early, curable stage. In the days of my residency training more than 25 years ago at the Mayo Clinic, we blindly used our fingertip to direct biopsies of the prostate. This was fine at the time, because it was all we had. Many cancers were missed, simply because the technique was relatively crude, even in the best of hands. Now, with ultrasound guidance, we can better sample the prostate systematically and detect even tiny abnormalities and direct the biopsies right to them.

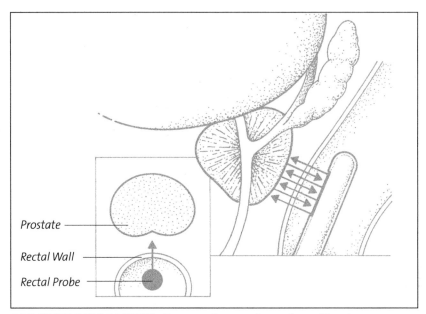

PROSTATE ULTRASOUND. Prostate ultrasound is performed by placing an ultrasound probe in the rectum, just behind the prostate. Sound waves are bounced into and off the prostate and surrounding tissues and reflected back to the probe. Closeness of the probe to the prostate itself allows for good visualization of the internal architecture.

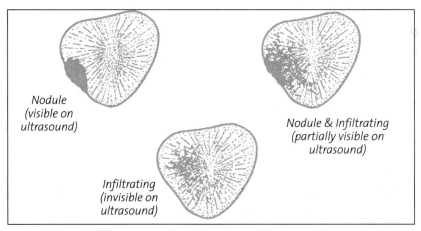

CANCER ON ULTRASOUND. Prostate ultrasound is best when trying to see large nodular cancers. Infiltrating prostate cancer that is evenly spread throughout the tissue may not be clearly visible on an ultrasound. Cancers that are a combination of both may appear to be much smaller than their actual size.

How is a prostate ultrasound done?

A lubricated ultrasound probe is gently inserted into the rectum. Sound waves are emitted from the end of the probe. They bounce off the prostate and are detected by the probe. These sound waves bounce at different amounts off different tissues, and are computer-generated into a picture. This allows your doctor to see the entire prostate on a small screen.

Does the ultrasound of the prostate hurt?

It can be very uncomfortable initially when the probe is inserted into the rectum. The good news is that the rectal lining has no nerves. For some men, inserting the probe can be painful, especially if they have a scarred or very tight anal sphincter muscle. Men who have had hemorrhoids repaired in the past may have scarring that can prevent insertion of the probe. This pain is only momentary, lasting just a few seconds. To make it more comfortable, many urologists use anesthetic jelly to numb the anal sphincter and inject a local anesthetic solution into the tissues surrounding the prostate. I have found this added numbing gel and injection to be fast, safe and extremely helpful.

Afterward, most men say the procedure wasn't as bad as they had expected, although it clearly is not something they want to do again unless necessary.

Can I just have an ultrasound, or do I really need biopsies as well?

The ultrasound alone is not a good test, and is not done just to look at the prostate. Although it may show us definite areas of concern, at least 20% of the time cancer can be present but not seen on the ultrasound. This may reflect the machine's quality, a technical problem or a lack of experience by the doctor reviewing the scan.

Sometimes the type of prostate cancer can't be seen on the ultrasound scan. Whatever the reason, it is considered standard practice to do a series of ultrasound-directed biopsies even if the ultrasound appears normal. I like to look at the ultrasound as a scope on a rifle—it lets you focus on your target, but it doesn't capture the information needed.

Doctor's Note!

I saw a patient who was being cared for by a urologist and was concerned about cancer because of an irregularity on his prostate exam and a mildly elevated PSA. Once a year he saw his urologist who performed a routine ultrasound without any biopsies.

Each time no ultrasound abnormalities were seen. The urologist therefore assumed nothing was wrong and sent him home, with instructions to come back in one year.

After several years of this, I saw the patient for what had become a very high PSA and a very hard, abnormal prostate. We went ahead with an ultrasound and biopsies. The ultrasound was still normal, but the biopsies all came back with a very aggressive cancer. Subsequent testing showed the cancer had spread to his bones. The lesson: A normal ultrasound alone means nothing.

What if I had an ultrasound and I was told nothing was seen, but no biopsies were done?

I do not agree with this approach. If there is a level of concern because the PSA is elevated and/or there are definite abnormalities on the exam, then you need to have biopsies to obtain tissue samples. I think it is wrong to assume that a normal ultrasound means no cancer. In fact, I have had a number of patients with very aggressive cancers whose ultrasounds were completely normal.

Does it make a difference who does the ultrasound evaluation?

The ultrasound is most often done by the urologist at the time of the prostate biopsies. There are some institutions where a radiologist may help with the ultrasound portion of the study.

Do I have to worry that I'm being told to have a biopsy that I really don't need?

No. It is standard care to do an ultrasound with biopsies if there is an abnormal digital exam, a change in exam, increasing PSA, low free-to-total percentage PSA or an elevated PSA.

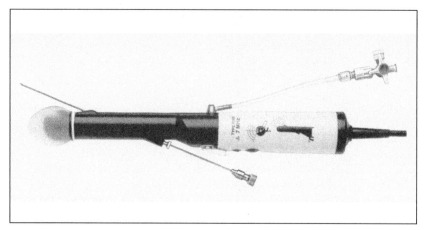

ULTRASOUND PROBE. This probe accurately directs sound waves into the prostate. The reflection (bouncing back) of the sound waves, depending on the different tissues, creates a picture of the entire prostate gland. Most probes allow the biopsies to be done directly through the probe, under ultrasound guidance. This allows for a quick, accurate sampling of the prostate. Photo courtesy of B and K Medical.

Is there any radiation exposure with ultrasound?

No, ultrasound uses harmless sound waves to generate a picture on the screen. Different tissues reflect sound waves differently, creating a picture of the inside of the body.

What does the probe do?

The probe not only emits sound waves in a certain pattern, but also receives reflected waves. The waves then are visible on the machine, forming the picture we see on the monitor.

Aren't there other ways to ultrasound the prostate than through the rectum?

Scanning through the abdomen doesn't provide the clear picture or allow for biopsies. Scanning the abdomen would allow for evaluation of the bladder, but not the prostate because of its location down deep behind the pubic bone.

What exactly is a prostate biopsy?

In a biopsy of the prostate, multiple tiny hairlike pieces of prostate tissue are obtained for microscopic analysis to see if cancer is present. These pieces are

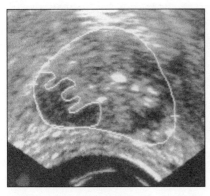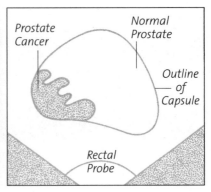

ULTRASOUND IMAGE. Ultrasound image at left is actually a continuous picture, with still photographs taken to document the findings. Here the cancer is
seen outlined as an irregular area of darkness. Biopsies confirmed this to be a rather
aggressive prostate cancer. Diagram at right clarifies what is shown on the ultrasound image.

obtained through a long, but very thin, needle, specially designed to open
up inside the prostate, take the sample, and then close.

Originally these tissue samples were all taken by hand without anesthesia, which was a slow and painful process. I was lucky if the patient would
allow me to obtain more than a few. I would often take men to surgery
and under a general anesthetic, with the patient asleep, perform the necessary biopsies.

Now a high-speed biopsy gun allows biopsies to be done with a much
smaller needle. Each biopsy can take just a few thousandths of a second.

For almost all men, biopsies can be done as an outpatient office procedure
without anesthesia and with usually only temporary discomfort. Now we
can get a good representative sampling of the entire gland with minimal
trauma to the gland.

What is a transrectal biopsy?

For a *transrectal* biopsy, the needle is inserted into the prostate through the
rectal wall. The rectal wall is thin, so it is possible to place the needle more
accurately and with less injury to other tissues. Because of its simplicity and
accuracy, this is by far the most common technique used.

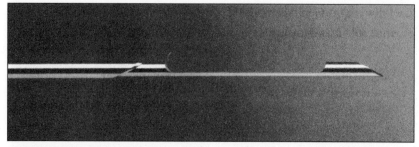

BIOPSY NEEDLE. New biopsy needles are small and very precise in removing tiny slivers of prostate tissue for microscopic analysis. This is a highly magnified view of a needle, which is only 1.2 mm in diameter. Closed needle enters tissue. Sheath slides open and closes onto a sample of tissue and the needle is withdrawn. Photo courtesy of C.R. Bard Inc.

What is a transperineal biopsy?

Another, less common, technique is what is called the *transperineal* biopsy. Instead of putting the needle through the rectal wall, the skin under the scrotum is numbed with a local anesthetic. The biopsies are then performed through this tissue, with less risk for infection.

This procedure is much less accurate and requires the needle to be placed through a more sensitive area of the body. Men prefer the transrectal approach.

Do I need sedation to relax me for the biopsies?

No. The procedure takes just a few minutes, and for most men it is momentarily unpleasant, so that sedation is not needed. Some doctors may use some degree of sedation. It is a personal preference.

Will I need a ride home?

Although it is not necessary, I usually ask that you have a ride home arranged just in case you are uncomfortable. You may be sore and distracted by the discomfort, so it is best if someone else can drive you home safely.

Can I play golf or tennis the next day?

Yes. There should be no real limits on your activity the following day.

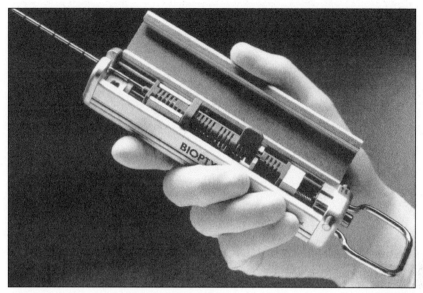

BIOPSY GUN. Spring-loaded, handheld biopsy gun allows very rapid and accurate removal of prostate biopsies in just a few thousandths of a second. Photo courtesy of C.R. Bard Inc.

How soon can I drink alcohol after the biopsy?

Hold off on alcohol for a few days until all the antibiotics you were provided have been taken. This is to prevent any potential interaction between alcohol and drugs. In addition, alcohol can sometimes increase the risks for urination difficulties after a biopsy.

How many biopsies need to be done?

Most men should have on average between at least eight to twelve to fourteen separate biopsies at the time of the procedure to get an adequate sampling of the gland (four to seven biopsies on each side). Experts now call for additional biopsies of areas along the outer margins and apex (tip of the prostate), where some cancers can be present and occasionally missed.

If specific areas of concern are seen, or if there is a definite nodule found on digital exam, then biopsies should also be directed to these spots. Sometimes, finger-guided biopsies will be done as well as ultrasound-guided biopsies. The

?

Does having a biopsy enable cancer to spread?

No. There is no evidence that cancer spreads simply because of
the biopsy. Though it might seem like doing a biopsy could
release cancer cells into the system, this does not happen.

average number is between eight and twelve, although some urologists do
more, others less.

What are the risks of a prostate biopsy?
The main risks are bleeding and infection. These are quite rare, occurring in
less than one in a hundred men. But it is important to be aware so that if
you have any concerns afterward, you'll be able to notify your doctor early
on and take appropriate steps to prevent serious problems.

How likely is it there will be bleeding afterward?
Some bleeding after prostate biopsies is very common and in fact expected.
This is because the needle passes through the rectal wall and into the prostate
gland, which can be surrounded by many veins. This is why I tell my patients
that they should expect to see blood in their urine, semen, and with bowel
movements, on and off, sometimes up to a few weeks.

Occasionally, blood can be seen in the semen for a few months after a
prostate biopsy. This is expected and should not cause you to worry. We are
concerned only if the bleeding is heavy and prolonged, as it can lead to difficulty urinating, requiring placement of a catheter or—very rarely—surgery
under anesthesia to find the bleeding spot.

If there is blood in the semen, does that mean cancer cells are present?
No. Blood in the semen is a direct result of taking tiny slices of tissue with
the biopsy needle. Occasionally, there will be bleeding into the seminal vesicles or into the prostate. When these glands then secrete the fluid during

ejaculation, blood may be seen. There is no relationship between blood in the semen and whether or not cancer is present.

How can a biopsy cause an infection?

Infection can occur because of the introduction of the needle through the rectal wall into the prostate gland. With appropriate antibiotic preparation and antibiotics afterward, infection is very rare. Rarely, tiny amounts of germs can be taken into the gland and can result in the development of an infection of the prostate and urinary tract.

Even more uncommon is an infection in the bloodstream, with high fevers and shaking chills, called *sepsis*. This can be quite serious and needs urgent medical attention! If you develop high fevers, you most likely will need hospitalization and powerful antibiotics. You must call your doctor or go to the nearest emergency room immediately. This is more common in men with a prior history of prostate infection.

How common are these risks?

Fortunately, these serious side effects are quite rare. Most men are surprised by just how well they did. I call my patients within a day or two to see how they are doing. Most say they are doing fine without any complaints.

What can be done to minimize the risk for bleeding?

To lower the chances of bleeding, you need to stop taking aspirin and aspirin-containing products for seven to ten days before the biopsy. You also should stop taking ibuprofen, Advil, Motrin, and other non-Tylenol pain and anti-inflammatory medications three days before a biopsy. If you are unsure what you should or shouldn't take, ask your doctor first. Also see the anti-inflammatory medications list on page 178. You should stop taking vitamin E, fish oil tablets and garlic supplements several weeks before the biopsy because these are all mild blood thinners.

Why won't my doctor do the biopsies if I'm taking aspirin?

Aspirin keeps normal clotting mechanisms from working. It blocks the blood product called *platelets* from functioning and from stopping bleeding. This means you can have an increased risk of bleeding.

How long in advance do I have to stop taking aspirin before the
biopsies are done?
I ask my patients not to take aspirin for ten days before biopsies. If there is
a good reason to stay on aspirin, I will do biopsies if the patient is off aspirin
for five days with the understanding of rare but possible increased bleeding
risk. This should be coordinated with your doctor.

Why won't my doctor do a biopsy if I'm on Coumadin blood thinner?
Coumadin acts to thin the blood so it won't clot and stop bleeding. If you
cut or scrape yourself while taking Coumadin, you will bleed much more
than if you were not on the blood thinner.

To biopsy the prostate of a patient on Coumadin would increase the risk
of severe bleeding. This bleeding can be quite significant and even require
hospitalization or surgery to control.

If you need a biopsy, you will need to be taken off Coumadin by your cardiologist and/or primary-care doctor. I prefer to get permission from all your
doctors before I ask you to stop important medications such as Coumadin.
You may be told to check blood levels just prior to the biopsy.

What options do I have if I'm on Coumadin and have an abnormal
prostate exam or PSA test?
You could stop the Coumadin and have the biopsies, or you may want to repeat the PSA test and digital exam in four to six months. If there is not a
dramatic change in the PSA test or digital exam, you might be able to postpone a biopsy and thus avoid the risks of stopping the blood thinner. For
some men, the risk involved in stopping blood thinners is high, so we either
watch them closely or consider treating them conservatively.

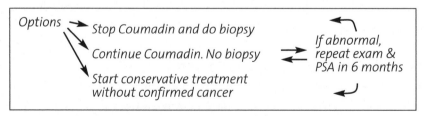

Suspicious exam with elevated PSA—Patient on Coumadin blood thinner.

What is done to stop the bleeding from a biopsy?

For heavy bleeding in the urine, under anesthesia, the urologist might perform a cystoscopy (look inside the urethra and bladder) and cauterize any bleeding spots. If severe rectal bleeding were observed (which I have never seen), the bleeding source would have to be located and cauterized by a gastroenterologist (GI specialist).

Can anything be done to stop the bleeding without surgery?

In the vast majority of biopsies, the bleeding will stop on its own. To help this along, I ask you to drink lots of fluids to flush out any blood and to avoid strenuous activity. You should avoid sex or becoming constipated. Both can prolong bleeding.

What can I do to prevent infection?

To reduce the risks of infection, we first make sure you do not have an infection at the time of the biopsy. We check the urine for bacteria or white blood cells, the cells your body uses to fight infection. We also give you antibiotics to take by mouth before the biopsy and for several days afterward. Many urologists will also give you an injection at the time of the biopsy to be sure that antibiotics are at a peak level in the tissues and bloodstream.

Can any other problems develop?

Very rarely, if there is a significant blockage, one can have swelling of the prostate gland and have difficulty urinating. This can result in urinary retention, which means you would be totally unable to urinate and your bladder would continue to fill and fill. This is very painful. It requires placement of a small rubber tube, called a *catheter*, to allow urine to drain out. How long it stays in depends on a number of factors, including how much urine is in your bladder when the catheter is placed. If you have trouble urinating, you should call your urologist immediately.

Can I become impotent after a prostate biopsy?

This is extremely rare, and I have only seen this once. It would be quite rare to have enough significant inflammation and swelling on both sides of the prostate to impact on erections.

After a biopsy some patients have expressed concerns and fears about ejaculation, pain, and bleeding that could potentially impact on erections from a psychological point of view.

Do the ultrasound and biopsy hurt?

Not for most people. It is uncomfortable to have the ultrasound probe placed, and the biopsies can sting a bit. The biopsy feels similar to a rubber band being snapped against the skin, just inside the rectum. Usually the first few biopsies are tolerated well. The last few can become more uncomfortable and even a little painful. Some men describe a cramping sensation that usually passes in a few minutes. I am always pleasantly surprised when most patients say afterward that it wasn't as bad as they had anticipated.

What if my doctor just wants to do a finger-guided biopsy without the ultrasound?

This would be rare. If the biopsy is done away from my office, and no ultrasound machine is available, then the only way to do a quick biopsy may be finger-guided. In general, though, I think it is much better to have biopsies with ultrasound guidance.

Who analyzes the tissue samples?

The slivers of prostate tissue (cores) are sent to be prepared and analyzed by a pathologist, a doctor who is trained in analyzing tissues, who will look at the tissue under a high-power microscope to see if malignant cells are present. Often, the slides will actually be seen by several pathologists, who must all agree before a report is issued. If there are any questions, the tissue slides can be sent to another group of outside pathologists who may have more extensive experience.

How long does it take to get biopsy results back?

On average, it takes about 48 hours for most labs to get results to my office. Some pathologists can have results back in 24 hours, while others may take five to seven or more days to process the specimens and generate a report. If the pathologist is out of town at an outside lab, then extra delays are common. Some outside labs, though, will process specimens and fax or call the result back to the office. Weekends and holidays slow down everything.

Is there a chance that someone else's specimens will get mixed up with mine in the lab?
Extraordinary measures are taken to be sure that what the urologist sends to the lab is accurately identified.

Should I have tissue specimens sent out for a second opinion?
If you or your doctor have any concerns, a second opinion is a good idea. The glass slides that have the tiny slivers of tissue can be sent anywhere in the world, but it may cost you several hundred dollars that might not be covered by your insurance plan. Sometimes even the pathologist will have additional questions and will send the slides out for additional opinions. I often direct second opinions to labs that specialize in analyzing prostate biopsy slides. The extra few hundred dollars is well worth the added peace of mind and confidence in the pathology report, and is usually paid for by Medicare or your insurance. Because the information from these slides is so important, I have always encouraged second opinions from specialty pathologists.

If the biopsies return showing no cancer, does that mean I don't have to worry?
No. Pathologists can only look at those tiny bits of tissue they are given to analyze. If a cancer is present in the prostate, but simply missed by the biopsy,

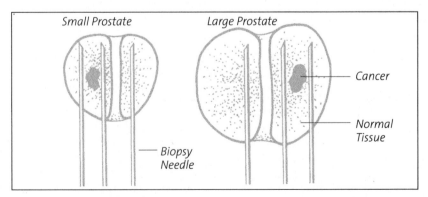

SAMPLING ERROR. Occurs when cancer is present but missed by the biopsies. It is easier to miss a cancer in a large prostate.

then naturally the report will come back negative, showing no cancer. This is called *sampling error*. There is no way one can safely and accurately biopsy every part of the prostate without removing the entire gland. Remember, the pathologist can only describe and evaluate what he or she is given. From that analysis, we try to project what is left behind. If there are any concerns, then you may need more biopsies in the future.

What if the pathologist isn't sure there is cancer?

Sometimes the pathologist doesn't have enough tissue to give a definitive answer, or the findings are suspicious. We don't want the pathologist to guess. When this happens, the pathologist will often recommend that you follow up with your urologist in two to three months and possibly repeat the biopsies. Again, it is easy and often helpful to send the specimens to a specialty pathologist who can often provide a more definitive answer.

What actually is written on the biopsy report?

The prostate biopsy report describes how much cancer is seen and how aggressive (grade) it is. Is it invasive into surrounding tissues or is it just a little

If I have had a biopsy that shows no cancer, what are the odds cancer is present but was simply missed by the biopsy samples?

A small but significant percentage—about 15–25%—of men with a negative biopsy still have cancer of the prostate and may need repeat biopsies and close, regular follow-up. This depends on the skill and experience of the urologist and where the biopsies were taken from within the prostate. If you have an abnormal exam and an elevated PSA with a negative biopsy, you must at least be followed closely. Many experts now suggest that all biopsies that don't find cancer should be followed by a second biopsy several months later. Some doctors use the PCA3 test to help decide how suspicious they are and whether or not to repeat the biopsies or follow the PSA level and exam closely.

speck? From this report, we try to estimate the true clinical picture. We take into account the PSA level, past PSA levels, the exam, family history and symptoms to predict your situation, and what treatment options are best for you.

The amount of cancer seen on the biopsies measured as a percentage of each core of tissue is important. Some experts believe this is useful to predict the volume of cancer in the prostate.

What are understaging and overstaging?

Understaging refers to a situation when the amount of cancer in the biopsy is not an accurate reflection of how much cancer is really in the prostate. If the biopsy shows a tiny amount of cancer yet there is a large volume in the prostate, then you will be understaged, and your doctors will assume you have far less cancer to deal with than you really do. Overstaging is when the biopsy shows a lot of cancer but there really is only a small amount in the prostate. Here your doctors will incorrectly think they are dealing with a large volume of cancer. This is far less common.

I have seen cases where the entire gland was filled with cancer, from right to left, front to back, and yet the initial biopsy showed only a small speck of low-grade cancer. This confirms what we all know—that a small volume of cancer seen on the biopsy may not be an accurate predictor of the actual volume of cancer in the prostate. Usually when there is extensive cancer in the biopsy, the prostate contains abundant cancer, but this is not always the case. Location of the cancer may be important to your doctors as well.

How often is cancer reported when none is really there?

Some of the world's leading prostate cancer pathologists have reported that the rate of false positives (cancer reported when no cancer is present) is 1 to 2 per 100 reviewed. This is another great reason to get a second opinion.

What is a saturation biopsy?

When your doctors remain highly suspicious that you have a cancer but none is seen on biopsies, a *saturation biopsy* may be suggested. A saturation biopsy involves performing many more cores than normally would be obtained.

This usually requires sedation or anesthesia. A saturation biopsy can increase the chances of finding a cancer, but again may miss one as well.

What will it cost to analyze the prostate tissue?

Cost depends a great deal on where the specimens are processed. It is almost always covered by insurance or Medicare. If the pathologist who performs the analysis is in a big city, it can cost quite a bit more than if the laboratory is in a smaller, more rural area. Also, the number of specimens sent out will affect the cost. The cost can range from about several hundred dollars to over $1,000 or even more. A second opinion will only cost $250 to $400 on average.

What does it cost to have a prostate ultrasound with biopsies?

The charges can range from $450 to $1,500, depending on where the study is done (hospitals are more expensive) and who is involved. If a radiologist participates with the urologist, fees can be higher. As with most medical services, what the doctors can charge is dictated by Medicare and insurance companies.

Why does it cost so much?

You are being charged for use of expensive high-tech ultrasound equipment, which can cost well over $100,000. You also pay for the disposable biopsy needle, use of a $1,500 biopsy gun, the urologist's time, skill and expertise in interpreting the ultrasound pictures, and the knowledge of where to direct the biopsies.

What about contrast-enhanced color Doppler, or 3-D prostate ultrasound?

These are new ways of performing the ultrasound and studies suggest they may add additional information and increase the chances of detecting a cancer. These machines are fairly new, require more expertise and are very expensive. Some of the newer black-and-white machines offer much better images than the older models. Even the best machine is limited by the skill and expertise of the operator.

NO CANCER IS FOUND— AM I IN THE CLEAR?

9

After you've had a prostate biopsy, the absolute best news is that no cancer was detected. However, no test is 100%, and there can be times when repeat biopsies may be needed. There is always a chance the first biopsy could have missed a cancer present somewhere in the prostate gland given that, even in the best of hands, prostate biopsies are a partial sampling process. Depending on how concerned your doctor is, you should probably talk to your urologist about a PCA3 test and a repeat rectal exam and PSA blood test in four to six months. It is your responsibility to ask and arrange for follow-up.

What is sampling error?
When cancer is actually present, but the biopsies do not find it, we call that *sampling error*. This happens because the needles missed the cancer within the prostate! This detection error occurs about 15–25% of the time. Because of the possibility of sampling error, we can only say that we do not find any cancer in the biopsied tissue. We can't completely rule out the possibility of cancer. For this reason, it is essential that you continue to see your urologist regularly.

Does a negative biopsy mean I don't have cancer?

No. It only tells us that no cancer was seen in the tissue analyzed.

Does the repeat biopsy, the second or third time around, ever show cancer?

Yes, occasionally it does. The more biopsies you have that are normal, the less likely that additional biopsies will show anything. The good news is that cancers found on subsequent biopsies tend to be smaller and less aggressive.

Should I have repeat biopsies?

This depends on the level of suspicion and the trend of PSA levels over time. If the biopsies return as normal with no cancer seen, and your doctor is very suspicious that there may be cancer present, he or she may want to repeat the biopsies in a few months. Your doctor may believe there is a good chance cancer is in the prostate but that it was missed with previous biopsies. If your digital rectal exam continues to change, the PCA3 is abnormal, or if the PSA level continues to rise, then he may also want to repeat the biopsies.

The first round of biopsies will detect up to 80% of cancers. If you go back for a second pass, there is a 13–20% chance of detecting a cancer. Sometimes we need to do more than two sets of biopsies. The most I have ever done to a patient is five separate sets of biopsies, over a several-year period. That patient had an abnormal prostate nodule, and his PSA level was increasing. We ultimately did find cancer, which was treated successfully.

I saw a young man with very advanced prostate cancer and a PSA of more than 250. We talked and reviewed his records. Unfortunately, several years before he had undergone an ultrasound and biopsy for an elevated PSA of 9, which came back normal. Although he was told to return to be rechecked in four months, he decided it wasn't necessary and in fact moved to another city in the meantime. It can't be emphasized enough: Even a "clean" or normal biopsy can miss a cancer, and regular follow-ups and monitoring of the PSA and exam are needed, sometimes with repeat biopsies.

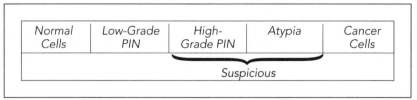

Normal Cells	Low-Grade PIN	High-Grade PIN	Atypia	Cancer Cells
		Suspicious		

PIN. Normal cells can turn into very low-grade changes called low-grade PIN. High-grade PIN is a suspicious premalignant change. Atypia is even more worrisome. Finding high-grade PIN or atypia on a biopsy raises serious concerns about cancer adjacent to the tissue biopsied, requiring close follow-up and probably repeat biopsies.

How should I be monitored after the biopsies if the report comes back fine?

It depends on your age and the level of concern you and your doctor have. Most often, I recommend a recheck of the PSA level in about four to six months. If the PSA level is about the same, then I would repeat it six months later. If it is still unchanged, then probably a repeat test every six or twelve months would be fine. Again, if I have concerns, a PCA3 test may add information.

What if they find PIN on the biopsies?

PIN stands for *prostatic intraepithelial neoplasia*. This term is used by pathologists to describe suspicious, abnormal areas seen on biopsied tissue. These areas are not cancer, but they are not normal either. High-grade PIN and prostate cancer are related but how remains uncertain. The significance remains controversial.

High-grade PIN should be considered a premalignant or precancerous change at the least. Experts consider high-grade PIN as a potential marker of significant prostate cancer, often requiring a second round of biopsies. High-grade PIN may also be found adjacent to cancer, suggesting that the biopsies were very close but just missed hitting a cancer in the prostate.

What is atypia?

Atypia on biopsies is a term used to describe abnormal cells that have some findings that look cancerous but not enough to be called prostate cancer. This is even more of a concern than PIN.

What should I do if I have high-grade PIN or atypia identified on biopsies?

If you have high-grade PIN or atypia on a biopsy, then you probably need a second round of biopsies, with special attention to the sides and apex of the prostate, where cancers can easily be missed.

If I have high-grade PIN or atypia, why can't I just go ahead and have surgery or radiation?

Even though this is often related to cancers, I believe that high-grade PIN or atypia itself is not a threat. Plus, inflammation or irritation of the prostate can cause changes that look like atypia. Therefore, it would be inappropriate and too aggressive to treat you just for these suspicious changes. If we identify a true cancer, then we can talk about curative treatment options. High-grade PIN is not cancer, and though highly suspicious for adjacent or developing prostate cancer, the PIN itself does not need treatment. The finding of high-grade PIN or atypia should be followed closely with repeat biopsies. If they are negative for cancer, then we closely monitor the digital exam and PCA3, free-to-total and complexed PSA and consider additional biopsies in the future. There are some experts who do think that treatment for significant atypia may be reasonable.

How could my doctor have missed biopsying a cancer if it is present?

Many cancers are present in small clusters or may be limited to a hard-to-reach region. Biopsies must be directed to these outside regions, where the cancers "hide," as well as to the apex of the gland. Some doctors seek better results by varying the location of the biopsies or increasing the number of samples taken. It seems the location of the biopsies is as important as the number taken.

Are there any new tests to help identify cancer on biopsies?

Yes. One example is that when early prostate cancer antigen (EPCA) is seen on noncancerous tissue, we know there is a good chance cancer will be diagnosed in the future.

CANCER IS DETECTED—THE IMPORTANCE OF VOLUME

10

P robably nothing is more devastating than to be told that you have a cancer. In our society, the word *cancer* is associated with horrible treatments and death. Being told you have cancer can force you to look at your life and mortality in ways that you've never done before. But before you start thinking about the type of marble for your headstone, you should realize that most men will not die from their prostate cancer.

When cancer is detected in biopsied tissue, the challenge is to make an educated guess about how much cancer is in the prostate. This is done by looking at the few tiny slivers of tissue that we have examined. Your urologist must look at the big picture, taking into account the PSA, trends in the PSA levels over time, how suspicious the exam is, family history and any other signs or symptoms.

With this information, your doctor will decide which additional tests and studies are needed. These will depend on your age, health, PSA results and the specifics of the biopsy tests. Then you and your doctor can discuss the treatment options and decide what to do next.

Will the cancer kill me?

Probably not. This is not a time to panic—it's a time to gather information. Whether or not this cancer will be significant and affect the quality or length of your life depends on a number of factors. Further tests may be necessary to help your doctor decide if this cancer is a threat and how best to respond.

Does the amount of cancer in the biopsies tell us how much cancer is in the prostate?

It is a clue as to how much cancer is in the prostate, but no one considers it to be an accurate measure. This is, however, the only tissue information available. A small volume of cancer on the biopsy doesn't mean there is only a small cancer in the prostate. A large volume on the biopsy is usually an accurate reflection of a large cancer.

In my experience, there is usually *more* cancer in the prostate than we would guess from the biopsy report. We know this from looking at specimens removed during surgery and comparing them with the presurgery biopsy results.

What is tumor volume?

Tumor volume is the term used to describe how much cancer is present in the prostate. The more there is, the more aggressive the cancers tend to be, and the more concerned we become. We usually refer to tumor volume in cubic centimeters.

When I told Harlan, a 56-year-old train engineer, that we had found some cancer on the biopsy, he said, "Well, doc, I guess this is the end of the line for me." Without hesitating, I said, "No, Harlan, this isn't the end of the line. Now that we've found the cancer, we're just going to get off the train for a short time to fix this so you can get back on and continue your long and happy journey through life." Now, several years after treatment, Harlan is healthy, strong and continuing his journey.

Tumor volume is initially estimated based on the examination, PSA level, ultrasound and biopsy results. The only accurate way to measure tumor volume is after the prostate is removed and the pathologist can measure the size of the cancer.

Tumor volume is an important factor in determining the prognosis and options available for managing your prostate cancer. The larger and more aggressive it is, the greater the risks that it has started to grow outside the prostate.

THE GRADE OF CANCER— HOW BAD IS IT?

11

T he *grade* of a cancer is perhaps the single most important factor in predicting long-term results, response to treatments and survival. To describe the degree of a cancer's malignancy, we refer to its grade, which
is a standardized measurement. As with most cancers that can occur elsewhere in the body, there are various grades of prostate cancer.

The worst cancers are very aggressive, with the cells looking nothing like
original tissues. These are called *high-grade*, or *poorly differentiated*. Other
cells may resemble normal cells except for a few key points. These are called
low-grade, or *well-differentiated*. Some more middle-of-the-road cells are
called *intermediate*, or *moderately differentiated*.

Does the grade mean the same thing to all doctors?
Most pathologists and urologists use a special grading scale to help make
prostate-cancer evaluation more standardized. This way, two doctors across
the country can talk about a patient and both will understand the grade of
cancer in question. This also allows for a standardized approach to evaluating
and treating patients around the world.

Unfortunately, pathologists who specialize in prostate cancer can disagree
up to 50% of the time with the grading of the cancer by general pathologists.

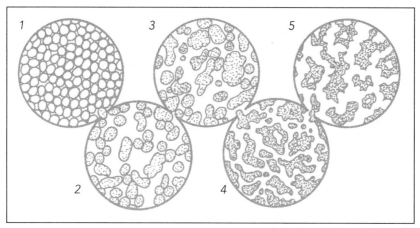

GRADE OF CANCER/GLEASON SCALE. The Gleason grading system is a standardized method of determining the grade of cancer. This technique utilizes cell shape and arrangements as part of the score.

Most general pathologists undergrade (rate the cancer less aggressive than it really is) but some overgrade the cancer (rate it as more aggressive than it really is). There are still concerns about this variability and how it may impact decision making.

How do you use the Gleason grade of cancer?

Like using cancer volume and the PSA level, the grade of cancer is an important indicator. In fact, all three are related. Larger cancers and higher PSA levels usually equate to more aggressive cancer cells. Left untreated, the cancer will continue to grow. As it grows it will secrete more PSA, and the cells will become more aggressive. Like a snowball rolling downhill, the cancer grows faster and faster. Many experts consider the grade to be the single most important factor in predicting how the cancer will respond to treatment and long-term results.

The rapid development of the cancer is why it is important to learn as much as possible by using the PSA test, prostate exam, ultrasound findings and biopsy results to decide what to do and when to do it. Ideally, we can use this information to cure you of your cancer during the window of opportunity.

What is the "Gleason scale"?

The most common grading scale for the comparison of cancers is the Gleason scale. In this grading system, cancer cells are assigned a certain point value based on well-accepted standard criteria. These criteria describe and rate the cancer cells in two ways: (1) how the cancer cells look and (2) how they are arranged together. Each component is given a number from 1 to 5, with the two numbers added together as the Gleason sum. Your urologist may refer to a cancer as a Gleason 7 or simply a grade 7. The higher the combined number, the worse the cancer. It is often reported as 3+4=7. The percentage of each grade is important.

What is the window of opportunity?

This is the time from the point of discovery of cancer until the time when the cancer begins to spread outside the prostate (see diagram on next page). During this time, you have more options to choose from, including choices that are potentially curative, such as radiation and surgery. When the cancer grows *outside* the prostate, options available will focus on cancer *control* rather than *cure*.

What is a low-grade cancer?

Low-grade prostate cancer is the least-dangerous type. Cancer cells look the most like the normal cells from which they came. They tend to be slow growing. They can be called *well differentiated*. On the Gleason scoring system, low-grade cells would be a 2, 3 or 4. This is the cancer to have. Probably this is what the more aggressive cancers started as, before they had time to grow and enlarge.

What is a high-grade cancer?

These cancers are the least like normal prostate cells. In fact, some can be so wild and aggressive that the pathologist might not even be able to tell what the original cell type was. These high-grade cancers are rapid growing, very

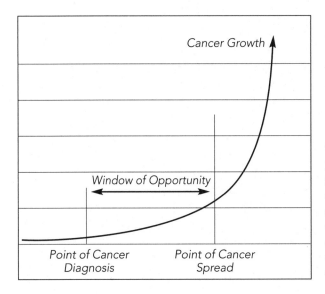

WINDOW OF OP-
PORTUNITY. The time
from when the cancer is
diagnosed until it has
started to spread is called
the *window of opportu-
nity*. During this time
curative treatments
should be successful.

aggressive and quick to grow into surrounding tissues. They can spread into the lymph nodes and bone.

High-grade cancers can be deadly. These are responsible for those rare stories of very rapid growth in relatively young men, such as the entertainers Bill Bixby and Frank Zappa. These cancers tend to be large. They are called *poorly differentiated* and are graded on the Gleason scale as the sum equaling 8, 9 and 10. High-grade cancers may be hard to treat and quick to come back. Some don't even respond to hormone therapy at all. The absolute worst are so wild that they may not even secrete the PSA enzyme, but this is rare.

How do the intermediate-grade cancers fit in?

As you might expect, they are somewhere in the middle, between the low-grade and high-grade cancers. Intermediate-grade cancer is what most men have when they are diagnosed with prostate cancer. These are called *moderately differentiated* and are graded as a sum of 5, 6 or 7 on the Gleason scale. These cancers can behave like either low-grade or high-grade cells, depending on how much tumor volume is present and how high the PSA is. A Gleason sum of 7 is considered to be a category by itself, more aggressive than 6, less than high-grade cancers. A cancer's aggressiveness is related to the percentage

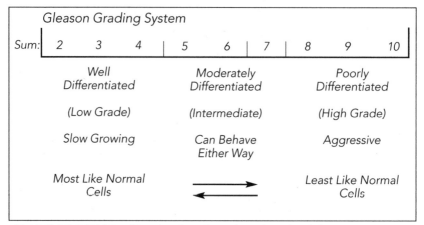

GRADE OF CANCER. Terms to describe each grade and its behavior are compared here with the Gleason system of grading cancer cells.

of the cancer that is grade 4 or 5, so the two numbers added together are important. For example, 3+4=7 is better than 4+3=7.

Do the cancers stay the same or do they always get worse?
Many are so slow growing that they may very well stay about the same over many years. Some, however, may reach that unknown critical mass where the volume gets so big that they begin to grow, becoming more aggressive and secreting more PSA into the bloodstream. It is thought that this volume of cancer may be about 1 cubic centimeter, or about the size of a cranberry. It may take 20 years or more of slow and steady growth to get this size.

What does perineural invasion on the biopsy mean?
Perineural invasion means that the cancer is starting to grow into small nerves, and this is a sign of aggressiveness. It is not invasion of the nerves that causes erections.

Does the grade of the biopsies tell what the grade of the cancer is in the prostate?
Most often, yes. We know that a surprising number of times we find that the final grade of cancer in the prostate is actually worse than what was biopsied and analyzed by the pathologists. I try to take this into account when counseling patients regarding the available options.

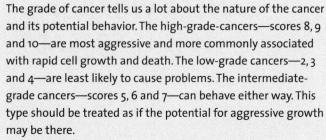

Why is the grade of cancer important?

The grade of cancer tells us a lot about the nature of the cancer and its potential behavior. The high-grade-cancers—scores 8, 9 and 10—are most aggressive and more commonly associated with rapid cell growth and death. The low-grade cancers—2, 3 and 4—are least likely to cause problems. The intermediate-grade cancers—scores 5, 6 and 7—can behave either way. This type should be treated as if the potential for aggressive growth may be there.

The Gleason score can be a valuable tool to help predict whether the cancer has not spread or may recur. I try to direct the treatment to the potential threat of the cancer, as suggested by the Gleason grade as well as the PSA, exam and stage. Stages are explained in Chapter 13.

Does the grade of cancer change over time?

Yes, as the cancer grows and becomes larger, it tends to become more aggressive. With prostate cancer, more advanced cancers tend to be largest, with the highest risk for spreading. This is why early detection can be so important.

What is "ploidy status"?

Ploidy status is a special study of the genetic material within prostate-cancer cells. This tells if the cancer cells are likely to respond to treatment. *Diploid* cancer cells are most likely to grow slowly and not spread. *Aneuploid* cells have the potential to behave aggressively and not respond as well to treatment. *Tetraploid* cells are somewhere in the middle. Most urologists have not found the ploidy status useful for discussing treatment options in most cases. In certain situations it can be a helpful tool.

Is there usually just one area of cancer in the prostate?

No. Studies show there are usually on average seven distinct and separate prostate cancers present. Each one may be a different grade, have a different volume and have a completely different potential for aggressiveness, growth and spread.

CANCER WORKUP— HAS IT SPREAD?

12

Y ou and your doctor will want to discuss treatment options after the diagnosis of prostate cancer. But first, your doctor needs to know whether or not the cancer has spread outside the prostate, and he or she also needs to determine the stage of the cancer.

Several tests are available to help us detect cancer outside the prostate, but none is perfect. This means a cancer could be present outside the prostate that is too small to be detected with current testing methods.

These tests provide valuable information about your cancer that will help us determine the most appropriate treatments. Whether or not we recommend a specific test depends on how suspicious we are that the cancer has grown outside the prostate and what information each test can provide.

Bone Scan

What is a bone scan?
A *bone scan* is a nuclear-medicine body-imaging technique where a tiny amount of radioactive substance is injected into the bloodstream. The substance circulates throughout the body and is absorbed by the bones. Certain

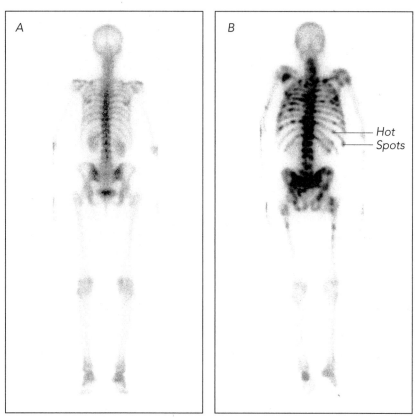

BONE SCAN. (A) Normal bone scan with no "hot spots" to suggest cancer spread to the bones. (B) Bone scan showing evidence of multiple areas where prostate cancer has spread and is growing in the bones.

abnormalities, including cancer, can be identified by this test. The substance then passes out of the body harmlessly.

The bone scan is the most sensitive imaging technique available today to identify cancer in the bones. The spine is the most common site outside of the pelvis for cancer growth. The scan often detects cancer in the bones long before regular X-rays can.

The bone scan doesn't show cancer, but it does show areas of rapid bone growth associated with cancer. Prostate cancer, when it spreads to the skeleton, typically has a classic pattern of random and variable *hot spots* that show up on the scan. Hot spots occur frequently along the spine, ribs and skull. For reasons we're not sure of, the arms and legs seem to avoid cancer's spread.

> **?**
>
> *My doctor has scheduled me for a bone scan. What is that used for?*
>
> The bone scan is used to detect whether the prostate cancer
> has spread. The spine and other bones are among the most
> common locations for the spread of prostate cancer.

The bone scan should be performed if the PSA is more than 10 and/or there is a high-grade cancer of concern. Sometimes if the PSA seems too low for the volume or grade of the concern, it is smart to check a bone scan.

Can anything else cause similar spots on the bone scan?

Other problems, cancerous and noncancerous, can also show up on the scan, but often with different patterns. It is the interpretation of these results that leads the radiologist to tell whether the images suggest the spread of prostate cancer, or some other process, or nothing at all. The report can only say whether the results look like cancer that has spread, which is referred to as *metastatic* cancer.

One of the most common irregularities is an old injury or fracture of a rib. Back surgery or a broken shoulder will show on a bone scan the same way a cancer would show.

Arthritis of the spine and bones and Paget's disease can also show on the bone scan. That's why it's important for your urologist to know your medical history so that he or she and the radiologist can best interpret the bone-scan results.

Can any other X-rays be done to see if the spots are from old injuries or broken bones?

You may need a few regular X-rays to see what the areas in question look like. If I am really concerned, I might order an *MRI scan* to look at the bone itself. This special scan, discussed in more detail later in this chapter, can let us get a better look inside the bones to see if it looks like cancer or not.

Morris seemed to understand his diagnosis of prostate cancer, and was eager to proceed with treatment. But he flatly refused to have the bone scan that was an important part of his evaluation. I wondered if this was his way of stalling because he just didn't want to have anything done, until his wife told me Morris was afraid the radiation from the scan would make his cancer grow faster. (He was embarrassed to tell me this himself.) Once I knew his concerns, we were able to communicate better.

Do you have questions or concerns of your own that you haven't mentioned to your doctor? Now, more than any other time, it is important to ask *all* of your questions, and keep asking until you fully understand your disease and your treatment options.

How can you tell if the spot on the bone scan is or isn't cancer?

If there is an area on the scan that does not look like it is caused by cancer, the radiologist will most often ask if you have had any injuries or fractures in that area. This way we can correlate any past history with irregularities on the bone scan.

So the bone scan can't prove for sure that cancer has spread?

No, it only gives us evidence that it *probably* has spread. This information is then reviewed together with the rest of the known facts to see if these findings are worrisome.

If the bone scan doesn't show anything, does that mean there is definitely no cancer spread to the bones?

No, it only means there are no cancer spots in the skeleton large enough to be detected by the equipment. There is no question that the equipment is very sensitive, but the cancer in bone marrow has to be present long enough, with enough increase in bone growth, to be seen on the scan. A negative bone scan is a fairly good indication that most likely there is no spread of cancer into the bones. A tiny cluster of just a few cells won't show up on the scan. This is the limitation to the study.

Even if I had an injury many years ago, it can show up on the bone scan?
Yes, sometimes old injuries show up even 50 or more years later.

Can't we just recheck the scan in a few months and see if it is growing?
Yes, this can be done if we really aren't sure. Most often, however, I use the test to help me determine what treatment options to recommend. Holding off a few months is not usually a good idea.

If it is cancer, is it always prostate cancer?
It probably is. There are several cancers that can spread to the bone. Prostate cancer is the most common. It would be very uncommon for a different cancer to show up on the bone scan when you are already known to have prostate cancer with a PSA level high enough to signal that spread to the bone is possible. Some other cancers that spread to bone include cancers of the breast (yes, even in men), bladder and colon.

What if there is only one spot on the bone scan, rather than the usual pattern?
Again, the radiologist would need to look at your past history and probably want to compare the bone scan with regular X-rays to see if there is evidence of an old injury. If there are still questions or concerns, an MRI scan can help to provide detailed information. Even then, if we're really uncertain, orthopedic surgeons can biopsy the bone and take out a piece of tissue for analysis.

What is a superscan?
In the usual bone scan, the kidneys show up as the radioactive substance is excreted. When there is so much widespread metastatic cancer that the kidneys don't even show up, this is called a *superscan*. This results because all of the radioactive material is going to the bones, so none is left to be filtered out of the blood by the kidneys. It is obviously not good to have so much cancer in the bones. This suggests a poor prognosis.

Does the bone scan hurt?

No. After the injection you wait an hour or so. Then you lie on a flat table and the imaging takes approximately a half hour.

What does a bone scan cost?

As with everything, much depends on where in the country you have the scan done. The price is about $2,500. Insurance and Medicare usually cover this expense, minus your deductibles.

Can I be admitted to the hospital to have this done?

No. It is an outpatient test that takes just a few hours and does not require you to be hospitalized.

Why is it always done at a hospital or in a big clinic?

The equipment used to perform the bone nuclear scan is quite large and relatively expensive, costing hundreds of thousands of dollars. It is not the kind of equipment that every doctor can have in his or her office. It is therefore usually based at a large facility that can generate enough testing volume to justify having it around. Some communities have the equipment brought in frequently on a large truck.

Will this hurt other organs or will I be radioactive afterward?

No. The amount of radioactivity injected is very tiny and will not hurt you or anyone else that you may be in close contact with.

If you fly cross-country a few times each year or live in a high-altitude community, you are exposed to more radiation on a yearly basis from background radiation in our atmosphere.

Will a bone scan increase my risks for getting other cancers?

No. There is no evidence to suggest that having a bone scan increases your risk of getting a new or different cancer later on.

Prostascint Scan

What is the Prostascint scan?

This scan is similar to a bone scan, but it looks primarily at soft tissues to see if the cancer may have spread. This is an elaborate test and may only be available in large cities or regional centers. This test is most helpful after radical surgery to identify the site of cancer recurrence. It can be a helpful tool when used correctly, though can be wrong up to 30% of the time. It can be difficult to interpret, even for an experienced radiologist. The results of the Prostascint test should be used with caution. Some have described the results as "disappointing." There are new versions with different markers, and these are promising.

CT Scan

What is a CT scan?

A *CT scan,* also called a *CAT scan,* which stands for *computerized axial tomography scan,* is a technique of evaluating the internal organs of the body with computerized X-ray pictures.

A machine revolves around you and generates a series of pictures. The computer then translates this information into pictures that look like cross-sections of your body. It is like being able to look at the internal organs without surgery.

X-rays are taken both *without* and then *with* dye in the veins to help identify blood vessels and internal structures. The intravenous dye can infrequently cause hives, itching and/or a warm sensation throughout your body. You usually also have to drink a shake of liquid dye to make the intestines visible. This liquid dye may cause diarrhea.

Rarely, a patient may experience a type of allergic reaction. If you have any allergies, you should notify the radiologist before you undergo the procedure.

For years, the CT scan was used routinely to help identify enlarged lymph nodes in the pelvis that might represent the spread of cancer. This usage has not turned out to be very effective. Most of the time, what we see with the CT scan doesn't provide accurate information regarding the lymph nodes. Sometimes the nodes will look fine, yet turn out to be full of cancer. Other

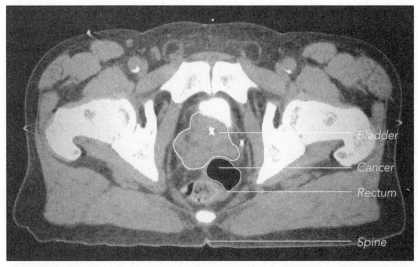

Bladder

Cancer

Rectum

Spine

CT SCAN. This scan shows a very advanced and enlarged prostate cancer with local growth into base of bladder, seminal vesicles and around the front of the rectum. Cancer outline includes prostate and cancer with seminal vesicles.

times, the nodes will look enlarged and suspicious with no cancer identified by the pathologist at the time of surgery.

Most urologists no longer order a CT scan before considering a radical prostatectomy. If you are going to choose radiation therapy for your cancer, then a CT scan is needed. The CT scan is used to help calculate how much radiation to deliver and where exactly in your body to deliver it.

What if my urologist wants me to have a CT scan before surgery?
There is always a small chance that something more serious than prostate cancer can be picked up by the CT scan, such as cancer of the pancreas or liver. If that were to happen, then there would be no reason to have prostate surgery.

If you are going to have to deal with a serious and life-threatening cancer other than prostate cancer, then you don't need to undergo the potentially serious side effects of prostate-cancer surgery. This is especially true if the prostate cancer will probably not be the dominant threat to your life.

In other words, as I often tell my patients, if you are driving down a steep mountain road and your brakes are failing, don't worry about whether or not the dome light works.

Will I be exposed to a lot of radiation?

No. There is more radiation with a CT scan than with a bone scan or even a chest X-ray, but it really isn't significant as long as you're not having one frequently.

Does the CT scan hurt?
No, not at all. You just lie on a flat table that slowly moves you through the inside of the CT scanner, which is like going through the middle of a giant doughnut.

What does a CT scan of the abdomen and pelvis cost?
The cost is quite variable but can be from $2,500 to $5,000 or more for a scan of the abdomen and pelvis.

MRI

What is an MRI?
MRI stands for *magnetic resonance imaging*. It creates high-quality pictures of the internal organs. Each molecule in your body has certain characteristics and responds differently to very powerful magnetic fields. When your body is exposed to these intense magnetic waves, the molecules that make up the cells give off specific amounts of energy. This energy is detected with sensitive scanners and computers to generate a cross-section image of the inside of the body. This result is similar to the CT scan, but MRI doesn't use X-rays.

Why did my doctor order an MRI after a bone scan wasn't clear about a spot?
The MRI has an advantage: It is excellent for looking into the internal makeup of bones and the spinal cord and brain. Sometimes an MRI can tell us if an abnormality in the bones is cancer or something else.

Is MRI useful for looking at prostate cancer?

Many urologists don't routinely order an MRI when trying to determine the stage of prostate cancer. MRI provides excellent pictures, but it may not tell us any additional information about lymph nodes or surrounding tissues that we can rely on. Some studies suggest that MRI could play an improved role if used with the rectal probe to better evaluate for spread of cancer outside the prostate.

Does an MRI hurt?

No. It requires you to be inside a long and narrow tube for the duration of the study. If you are claustrophobic, this may be a problem for you. Most men get over this in a few seconds, or they can take a mild relaxant before the test. The test can be quite loud, which is upsetting to some people.

What does an MRI cost?

About $3,000 to $4,000.

Why does my doctor want to do an MRI with a rectal probe?

Many experts believe that this special technique using an "endorectal coil" may provide additional information in the initial evaluation.

What is USPIO and how is it used with an MRI?

USPIO (ultrasmall superparamagnetic iron oxide) is a new and promising agent given 24 hours before the MRI to help light up prostate cancer cells. With this new technique, radiologists can now see bright spots that represent prostate cancer cells in the lymph nodes. This technique will be used for men who are at high risk for spread of prostate cancer, such as men having high PSA levels or very aggressive cancers.

What is a PET scan?

This new test, *Position emission tomography,* is like a CT scan but instead of looking at the internal structures of the body, PET scans look at areas of rapid cell growth.

Currently this test is not routinely used for prostate cancer, but it will probably have a bigger role in the future. The role of PET scan is evolving, especially for high-grade prostate cancer that has returned. A combined PET-CT scan is probably the newest test that will provide the most information.

STAGES OF PROSTATE CANCER

13

After all diagnostic tests are completed, your doctor can bring together all the information to make an educated guess about how much cancer is present and where it is located. This categorizing of the cancer helps us to identify treatment choices that are best for each particular stage.

When we talk about *how much* cancer is in a patient's body and exactly *where* it is located, we are referring to the *stage* of the cancer. The stage describes whether the cancer is small and confined to the prostate or large, with spread to any other tissues or organ, such as the bones.

How is the stage determined?
The stage is determined by information from the biopsies (for example, whether or not the cancer is on both sides of the prostate), the PSA level, the exam and any additional tests and studies that may be done.

What does the stage tell us about long-term results?
Basically, the more cancer in your body, the more potential for spread and the less effective the treatments are likely to be. The more aggressive the cancers are, as judged by the grade of the biopsy, the more likely the cancer will spread.

> ### STAGES OF PROSTATE CANCER
>
> Stage A   Cancer found incidentally or because of elevated PSA
> Stage B   Cancer found because of abnormal digital rectal
>   exam; cancer confined to prostate
> Stage C   Cancer spread to tissues outside of prostate
> Stage D   Cancer spread to lymph nodes or bone

Therefore, the worse the stage, the less optimistic we can honestly be about long-term results and survival. Some physicians would consider a worse stage as reason to hold off on aggressive treatments, because the treatments probably won't be effective. Others argue that if there is an aggressive cancer, it is best approached with an aggressive treatment if there is any chance for a successful therapy.

What are the stages of prostate cancer?

The classic system uses Stages A, B, C and D. We initially use a clinical stage to describe the cancers. That means we use whatever we know to tell us where we think the cancer is located, based on clinical tests and results of biopsies. We only have accurate information when the prostate has been removed and the pathology results are available, the *pathologic* stage.

What do the different stages mean?

Stage A: the cancer is found incidentally at surgery for prostate enlargement. This means that it was *not suspected* when the man went in to have his prostate hollowed out to enable him to urinate better. This finding used to happen 10% to 15% of the time, but now it is very rare. We would receive the final pathology report from the pathologist looking at the presumed nonmalignant tissue and see to our surprise that cancer was found. How much cancer and what grade it is divides Stage A further into Stages A1, A2 and A3.

Stage A1: usually low-grade disease in small volumes. This is most often the type of prostate cancer where we simply monitor your PSA results. Treatment is not usually required. Regular follow-up is a must, however.

Is it better to have one stage than another?

Definitely yes. It is always much better to have a small-volume, low-grade tumor than a larger, more advanced, high-grade cancer. The smaller it is, the less likely it will be able to spread.

Stage A2: the cancer is high-grade and aggressive or seen in more than a few small specks. If there is a lot of cancer, whatever the grade, it is A2. Men with Stage A2 are usually treated, because most often a significant cancer is indeed present and only a small piece was identified.

Stage A3: a cancer is identified because of an elevated PSA alone. Most often these cancers are substantial.

Stage B: the cancer is detected because of an irregularity or nodule found on the prostate exam. Usually the cancer is relatively small and most often confined to the prostate. Stage B is further divided into two categories.

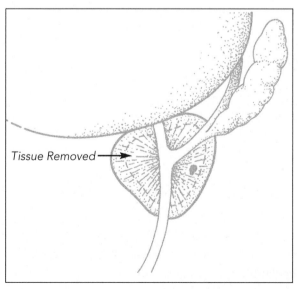

Tissue Removed

STAGE A1. Prostate cancer is described as Stage A1 when cancer is unsuspected and identified by the pathologist in the tissue removed following a transurethral prostate resection for blockage. The cancer should have a small volume and be low grade or intermediate grade.

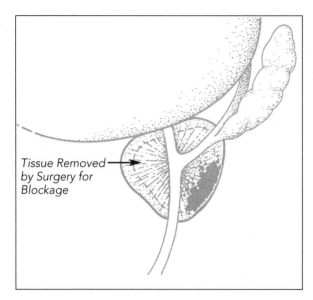

STAGE A2. Prostate cancers are also unsuspected and found during TURP surgery for blockage, but have higher-grade cancer and larger volume than Stage A1.

Tissue Removed by Surgery for Blockage

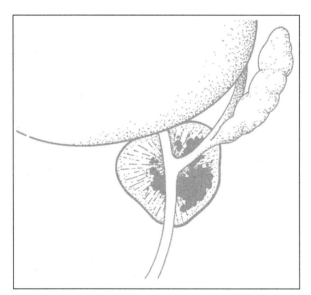

STAGE B. Cancer found by abnormal examination or elevation of the PSA that is still confined to the prostate gland is referred to as *Stage B.*

Stage B1: a prostate cancer located on just *one side* of the prostate.

Stage B2: the cancer is on *both sides* of the gland, but with no evidence of spread outside the gland or to bones or lymph nodes.

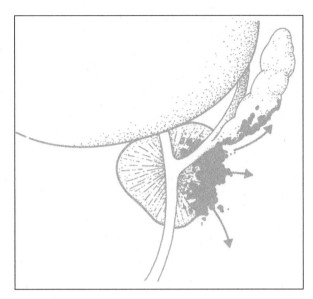

STAGE C. Cancer grow-
ing outside the prostate
gland and into surround-
ing fat, tissues and adjacent organs such as the
seminal vesicles is known
as Stage C.

Stage C: the cancer has started to grow *outside* of the gland, but with no spread
to bones or lymph nodes. It can be seen growing into the fat that surrounds
the prostate, or into the seminal vesicles or even into the base of the bladder.

Stage D: used to describe cancer that has spread either to lymph nodes or to
the bones.

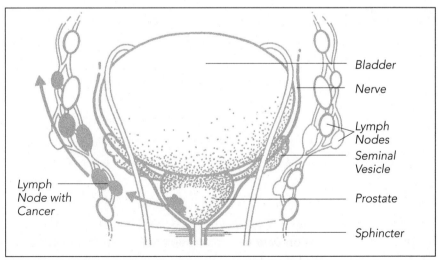

STAGE D1. Prostate cancer has grown outside of the prostate and traveled into the lymphatics and the lymph nodes of the pelvis.

Stage D1: indicates local spread of the cancer to the lymph nodes, confined within the pelvis.

Stage D2: the cancer has started to spread to the bones.

After surgery for prostate blockage (TURP, as explained in Chapter 1), how do you know if there is any cancer left behind when you only removed the core of the prostate?
We really don't know. If cancer is found in the tissues, then we need to decide if there is any cancer remaining. I have done prostate biopsies and a repeat TURP in the past. Now, I usually recommend that we follow the PSA levels if the amount of cancer is very small. If the amount is significant, then I recommend a more aggressive treatment for what we assume is cancer still remaining.

But my doctor said I was a "T2N0M0." Is that a different way of describing the stage of my cancer?
Your doctor is using the TNM grading system. This is an international system to replace the old A, B, C, D staging system. The TNM system is thought to be more accurate. It gives doctors worldwide a more standardized way of discussing and understanding the stage of a specific cancer case.

Does it make a difference which staging system my doctor uses?
No, as long as there is consistency between your doctor and other physicians involved with your case.

What does the T, N and M stand for?
T describes the cancer itself, with different numbers explaining how large the cancer is. *N* stands for nodes and tells us if the cancer has spread to the lymph nodes. *M* tells if the cancer has spread, or become metastatic.

Which system is better?
The TNM system is becoming more and more accepted around the world. Technically, it provides more specific information that everyone can use. This new system is slowly being adopted.

Comparison of the TNM and ABCD Staging Systems

TNM	ABCD	EXPLANATION
T1a	A1	Unsuspected cancer found incidentally during prostate removal (occupying less than 5% of prostate)
T1b	A2	Unsuspected cancer found incidentally during prostate removal (occupying more than 5% of prostate)
T1c	A3	Cancer that is detected only because of elevated PSA (normal exam)
T2a	B1	Cancer that is felt and occupies 50% or less of one side
T2b	B1	Cancer that is felt and occupies more than 50% of one side
T2c	B2	Cancer that is felt and occupies both sides of the prostate
T3a	C1	Cancer occupying one side and growing outside of the capsule
T3b	C1	Cancer occupying both sides and growing outside of the capsule
T3c	C2	Cancer that has invaded the seminal vesicles
T4a	C2	Cancer that involves the bladder neck and/or rectum and/or external sphincter
T4b	C2	Cancer that involves other areas near the prostate
N0	No equivalent	No cancer detected in the lymph nodes
N1 (N+)	D1	Cancer spread to one or more lymph nodes (2 cm of cancer or smaller)
N2 (N+)	D1	Cancer spread to one or more lymph nodes (2 to 5 cm of cancer)
N3 (N+)	D1	Cancer spread to one or more lymph nodes (5 cm of cancer or more)
M0	No equivalent	Cancer that is confined to the prostate, surrounding tissues and pelvic lymph nodes
M1 (M+)	D2	Cancer that has spread beyond the pelvic area to bones, lungs, etc.

What are the Partin tables?

These are probability tables developed by Dr. Alan Partin at Johns Hopkins Medical School to predict whether or not the cancer may have spread or may still be confined to the prostate. While this is a helpful tool, it should not be used to replace individualized review and recommendations based on the specifics of the individual case. If you have questions, ask your doctor.

Dr. Partin himself has told me that his tables were never intended to dictate which treatments a person should or shouldn't have. Rather, the tables are intended to provide additional information for consideration when making decisions regarding a person's care and treatment options.

What is the difference between clinical and pathologic stage?

The *clinical stage* is based on your examination, the PSA results, any X-ray results and the biopsy report. They are all suggestive of what is really going on. The *pathologic stage* is the actual stage based on the prostate tissue and lymph nodes removed.

What is T1C and why do some doctors not like the T1C category?

If the cancer was detected because of an elevated PSA alone, then this is staged T1C. Stage T1C unfortunately does not provide much information about the tumor itself. The cancer could be a very tiny, low-grade cancer or the prostate could be totally replaced by a very aggressive cancer.

FIVE CATEGORIES OF
TREATMENT OPTIONS

f you have been diagnosed with prostate cancer, the next major question is, "What can I do about it?" The reasons for each individual's treatment choice are different from person to person. What works for one man may not be an option for another. That is why it is important to understand the potential benefits and complications of each of the choices before you. Don't make any snap decisions based on emotion or incomplete information. Listen with an open mind, and then make your decision.

There are five categories of treatment from which to choose. Each category may include several options, and each choice has definite pros and cons. You should think carefully through each one to decide which is most appropriate for your particular situation.

It is impossible to decide what treatment is best for you based on the clinical stage of cancer alone. So many factors that cannot be addressed here must enter into your decision regarding treatment.

You should look at what the risks are up front and what the long-term risks and benefits are. The more risks you take today, the more potential for the best long-term results. Why is this so? Because in general, the more aggressive the treatment, the better the chances are for cure. And it is the aggressive treatments that have the potential for more risks to the patient.

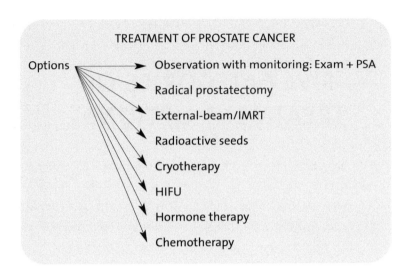

You must consider quality-of-life issues, your general health, family longevity and most basically, what scares you more—the cancer or the treatments.

The five basic treatment options:
1. Simple observation with monitoring of PSA levels.
2. Radical prostatectomy (abdominal, perineal or laparoscopic).
3. Radiation therapy (external-beam/IMRT or radioactive seeds).
4. Destructive therapies—cryotherapy (freezing the prostate gland) or HIFU.
5. Hormone therapy (monthly hormone injections or removal of the testicles) or chemotherapy.

Additionally, a number of alternative and integrative options are commonly discussed. (See Chapter 26.)

Which options fit into which stage classification of prostate cancer?
Stage A1 disease is where there is a small volume of low-grade cancer. The main treatment choices are between simple observation with close and regular follow-up (active surveillance) versus one of the curative options, such as radical prostatectomy or radiation therapy. (Radiation therapy is discussed in detail in Chapters 19 and 20; radical prostatectomy in Chapters 21 and 22.)

I look at the general health and age of the patient and try to get a feeling for how comfortable he is with no treatment. The large majority of men in this category will not die of their cancer even if nothing is done.

However, if you are young enough, in your 40s, 50s or early 60s, then you may live long enough for a small cancer to continue growing. The cancer might possibly lead to your death. Up to 15% of men who live long enough will die of the cancer if left untreated.

I routinely encourage my younger patients with prostate cancer to consider radical prostatectomy as the best long-term treatment. If they are not a candidate for surgery or choose not to have a prostatectomy, then radiation or radioactive seeds may be an effective second choice. Older men can decide on no treatment and monitoring of the PSA level.

Stage A2 is a different situation altogether. When a high-grade and aggressive cancer is found in the tissue removed during a TURP, we know it is likely that there is still a significant amount of cancer remaining in the prostate. In this case, aggressive treatment is warranted.

Men under 70 should consider having a radical prostatectomy. Men over 70 should have radiation, external-beam IMRT therapy (see Chapter 19) or radioactive seed implants (see Chapter 20). Only very old men in poor health should have no treatment or hormone therapy with close monitoring of their PSA level.

Stage A3/T1C is perhaps the most common stage, as men with normal exams are being found to have cancer simply because of an elevated PSA level. These cancers may or may not be cured by aggressive therapy. In this category, your age, general health, PSA level and the grade of the cancer may play a role in helping you decide which treatment is best. In more than 90% of the men, the cancers tend to be significant.

Stage B1 is the ideal stage for curative treatment. If you have a normal life expectancy of seven to ten years or more, then radical prostatectomy is probably the best first choice.

The cancer should be confined to the prostate, which means removing the gland would be curative. Radiation will also work well for B1 disease, both external beam and radioactive seeds. Observation may be acceptable if you are elderly and ill (by this, I mean in your 80s and with a limited life expectancy of just a few years).

Hormone therapy (discussed in Chapter 24) may be a reasonable option if you are older and not very healthy but want to have something done.

Stage B2 is also best treated with aggressive surgery or radiation. Some of these cancers will actually turn out to be Stage C, with some of the cancer outside the gland. A small percentage of Stage B2 patients may even have cancer in a lymph node.

If there is any question and you are young, I usually opt for surgery. If you are older (70 or older), then I may lean more toward radiation. The larger tumor volume tends to reduce the effectiveness of seeds. Because of the tumor volume seen in B2 disease, I am reluctant to just observe these cases, because if you live long enough, sooner or later these cancers will progress.

Again, hormone therapy may be reasonable if your life expectancy is less than five years and you want something done.

Stage C: My philosophy for men in their mid-60s and older is that these cancers are best managed with radiation therapy, because the radiation treatments often are focused on enough surrounding tissue to include any local spread. Stage C cancers are often quite large, which can make the radiation less effective. Occasionally the cancer cells may have already spread beyond the area treated by radiation.

I tend to give the benefit of the doubt to men in their early 60s and younger with Stage C disease. I usually suggest a prostatectomy on the possible chance that it may turn out to be curative. In fact, recent studies show that some men with large aggressive cancers can be cured with prostate removal. Simple observation is risky if you will live more than a few years. Hormone therapy may be fine for those with a limited expected life span of five years or less. Even if the surgery does not totally remove the cancer, then the addition of radiation or other treatments in a stepwise fashion is reasonable. This concept of combination step therapy is becoming more popular than the old thought of single treatment. Urologists used to ask, "What single therapy will give my patient the best chances for long-term survival?" Now we ask, "What series of treatments will be most effective?"

Stage D is when the cancer has spread outside the prostate, either into the lymph nodes, bone marrow or elsewhere. This stage is further divided into whether or not the cancer is confined within the pelvis (Stage D1) or appears outside the pelvis, as with bone involvement (Stage D2).

Treatment for this stage depends on the usual factors: age, general health and expected survival. I personally believe in early treatment of advanced disease, rather than waiting until the cancer is causing symptoms, as some physicians propose. Early treatment prolongs the time until the cancer comes back and may prolong the life span to some degree.

At this point we know of no effective cure for prostate cancer that has spread to the bones or lymph nodes. The treatment goal with Stage D is to control the cancer by eliminating the male hormones from the body. This is done because the male hormone stimulates the growth and spread of prostate cancer.

I agree with some experts who believe in *debulking*, or eliminating a lot of the cancer with radical surgery, even if it is clearly advanced. They believe that if the total volume of cancer in the body can be dramatically reduced by removing the prostate, the remaining small volume of cancer can be better controlled with hormone therapy. This philosophy is still debated. It may even be considered by some experts to be overly aggressive. Personally, I have seen some dramatic long-term results with this approach—adding hormone therapy to aggressive debulking of the prostate—in young men.

My philosophy is that for men in their early 60s or younger, if they are found to have a small volume of cancer in the lymph nodes at the time of node dissection, I may go ahead with the prostatectomy. My thinking is that the small speck or two in the nodes may be all there is, and perhaps there will be a chance for good long-term results. If instead we go ahead with hormone therapy alone, then there is no chance that long-term results will be as good.

In other words, for very young men, I tend to be aggressive in treatment with the thought that they have more to lose. There really is no second place in this race. In older men, I tend to be more conservative, because the risks

Ralph O., a general surgeon, saw me for a "second opinion." He brought with him an envelope filled with copies of records from eight other doctors he had seen for "second opinions" regarding what would be his best treatment option. Unfortunately, Ralph had completely exhausted and confused himself by gathering too much information. Without looking at any of the other recommendations, we sat together and started from the beginning, reviewing only his present health status and the findings of his tests—PSA, biopsy, bone scan. Together, we walked him through the options that were best for him, based on his disease, overall health, lifestyle and family background. By the time we finished, Ralph felt more in control and more confident in his ability to choose a treatment plan that would be best for him.

of the treatment go up with advancing age. It is important to consider the quality of life as well as longevity.

What should I do if the biopsies show very aggressive cancer, but the bone scan and CT scan are normal?

This is a topic of recent discussion among experts. With a high-grade cancer that is poorly differentiated (rapid growing), the odds are fairly good that the cancer has already spread outside the prostate, probably into the pelvic lymph nodes.

For very young, healthy men there is a chance that surgery may make a significant difference and could even be curative. There may be no evidence of spread of the cancer. In this situation, I would probably recommend the evaluation of the lymph nodes for cancer. If no cancer is seen, then I would go ahead with radical prostatectomy. Again, we can always add radiation treatment and chemotherapy. But for high-grade cancers, radiation tends to have a high failure rate.

***Should I consider just following an alternative diet instead of what
seems to be very aggressive treatments with potential risks?***
Absolutely not. Even the experts in alternative health would tell you to *integrate* the treatments. It's not a question of choosing one treatment instead of the other. First of all, many of the nutritional and alternative options have not been scientifically proven to help. But even if they had been, it's not wise to choose one option that may work, or even surgery or radiation alone. If an angry grizzly bear is charging you and you've got two rounds in your rifle, would you fire one shot and then throw down the gun? I believe in the power of using everything together. Fire both rounds and throw a rock at the bear! When dealing with a potentially life-threatening cancer, I encourage my patients to follow strict dietary changes and have the best standard treatment they can get. This way, they've done all they can do.

A sign in the office of Dr. Stephen Strum, a prostate cancer specialist in Oregon, reads: "Old Russian Sailing Proverb: Pray to God but don't stop rowing."

Remember that a potential risk doesn't mean it will happen for sure. In fact, most potential risks don't happen at all. That's why they're called *potential* risks.

WHO DECIDES ON TREATMENT—YOU OR THE DOCTOR?

15

When it is time to make decisions about cancer treatment, remember: You are in control. If you wish, you can choose to let your doctor make the decisions, or you can retain control and use your doctor as a resource of information and opinions. Who actually decides what to do varies with each patient and his doctors.

This area of discussion is usually left out when you are talking to your doctor. The usual scenario is for you to meet with your doctor so he or she can tell you what is wrong and what your doctor wants you to do. The review of options is brief and often biased toward whatever your doctor has decided is best for you.

Some physicians leave little time for your questions and concerns. Rarely are you encouraged to think about the various choices. A decision is almost always expected right then and there. In fact, sometimes the doctor goes so far as to schedule your treatment or surgery before you even arrive for your appointment.

Who decides what treatment option is best for me?

You should take an active role in deciding what you will do. For many years, the doctor knew what was best for his or her patients. He would proceed with the treatment without really involving the patient in decision making. Fortunately, those days are long gone.

Today, the doctor's role is to gather information necessary to provide a fair and reasonable review of the facts and present a detailed discussion of the treatment options. He or she should encourage you and your family to get involved in decisions. After all, you are the one who has to live with the outcome of the choice.

Ultimately, you are the one who must decide which treatment is best for you. You can give this power to your doctor, but again this is your choice. Whether or not your doctor agrees with your decision, your doctor should still be there to work with you and support you and your right to decide.

I must admit that for me, as a physician, it is sometimes very frustrating and upsetting to see a patient make what I believe to be a wrong decision. This is often the case when someone makes a final decision before he has all the facts, often after talking to a friend, relative or neighbor. In my experience, this is the absolute worst thing you can do.

You will hear lots of advice, horror stories and disasters, often having nothing to do with your specific situation. I can't tell you the number of times I've heard men refuse to consider radiation for prostate cancer because of what it did to Aunt Nellie after breast-cancer treatment 35 years ago.

Remember, the person giving the advice is basing the recommendations on his or her own personal experience or hearsay, not on actual statistics and the facts particular to your case. These friends usually know little if anything about your specific problem.

What if my doctor doesn't agree with my decision?
Be wary of the doctor who quickly shoots down what you believe to be a reasonable and acceptable option. Some doctors just aren't used to having someone disagree with them. There may even be other factors that enter into your doctor's recommendations. Ask your doctor why he doesn't agree with your choice. He or she may provide information you had not considered, or a different approach.

If your doctor will not respect your decision, you may need to find a doctor who will. However, in all fairness, there should be an open line of

> *Take an active role in deciding what you will do. For many years, the doctor knew what was best for his or her patients. He or she would proceed with the treatment without really involving the patient in decision making. Fortunately, those days are long gone.*

communication between you and your doctor. Be sure to listen to his or her reasons for not supporting you—they may be very legitimate.

Why do some doctors become angry when I tell them what I think is best for me?

Many patients make decisions based on incomplete or inaccurate information. This is extremely frustrating for the physician. I know one cancer specialist who jokingly says that all of his patients are cancer specialists. After all, they read a magazine article or a book! And who is he but a mere board-certified, highly trained, well-respected medical oncologist.

Although this is a bit sarcastic, it illustrates an important point. No matter what you've read (yes, even this book), your urologist is the one who deals with prostate cancer every day of every year. Your doctor's recommendations are based on personal experience, research studies, papers, books and the combined experiences of urologists around the world. Use this book and other resources as a basis for increasing your understanding.

How can I take back control?

By reading this book, you have taken the first step to understanding what we know and more importantly what we don't know about prostate cancer. Medicine is still more an art than a science. We treat individuals based on statistics gained from the cases of large numbers of men.

What works for many may not work for you. Ask questions and expect answers. Write them down. Talk to specialists. Talk to nurses. And when you have as much information as you need to make a decision, go ahead and choose the treatment you feel is best for you.

I recently had a 62-year-old man diagnosed with what I believed to be a potentially significant prostate cancer. After a complete consultation and initial moves toward a radical prostatectomy, he expressed an interest in trying a strict "anticancer" diet. This diet would best be described as nontraditional. I felt it probably wasn't going to work. But after a full discussion with my patient, I realized he truly understood what he was doing, and he knew the associated risks and possibility for cancer progression. I agreed to work with him and support his decision. Only time will tell if he made the right choice.

Don't let information gathering become your goal. And don't fall into the trap of deciding what you want the doctor to say and then start doctor-shopping until you locate one who will tell you what you want to hear. Listen to the answers. Listen to the questions your doctor asks you.

It is very important not to let the process carry you away. I've known a few patients who took up to six months to talk with expert after expert. Within a short time they were so confused and overwhelmed that they needed a break to just let it all sink in. Only then could they make a decision.

Should I try to keep my own medical records?

Yes. This is an excellent way to keep control over what is happening to you, in all aspects of your health. As you get PSA test results, record them on a log. See the Appendix for a Prostate Cancer Evaluation Log. Keep copies of your X-ray records, consultations, and so on. If something concerns you, then you have records for reference. Most doctors will be more than happy to send copies of your test results as they come in. Having records is also helpful when you travel. If you have a medical emergency in a different city, doctors treating you will know your past medical history and be able to take better care of you. I suggest that you take *copies* of your notes. If you should lose them, you still have the originals.

How do I decide which facts are important and which are not?
Again, this is where open communication with your doctor is essential. Too often men focus on the obscure or rare when making decisions. Be careful not to give unrealistic power to the various facts. Your doctor will help you, as will others in support groups or on the Internet.

One caution regarding the Internet: Everyone seems to have a strong opinion, and as a urologist I have a hard time separating the facts from the hype. When you read something on the Internet, ask yourself: Who wrote this? What are their credentials? Are they selling something? And finally, take everything with a grain of salt.

YOUR WIFE OR
PARTNER'S ROLE

16

Your wife may be even more devastated by the diagnosis of your prostate cancer than you are. She has been your partner, and she has pictured growing old with her life companion. Now, suddenly, this image may be challenged. So remember to include her in every step of decision-making. Ask her for opinions. Listen to her answers.

In the anxious excitement that follows diagnosis, it is not uncommon to forget to involve your wife or significant other in the long process of cancer evaluation, treatment, recovery and life after treatment.

Whatever path you choose, and no matter what happens, she will have to watch it from the sidelines. She will have to live with the results of your decision. It is sometimes easier to be the patient, because you are aware of what is happening every step of the way. From the first time you step into the urologist's office, through all the long appointments, tests, waiting for results, long discussions about treatment options and controversies, treatment, recovery period and then as you begin your life again—hopefully cured—there is your wife. She is often quietly sitting and waiting, trying to stay calm and support you while an almost overwhelming fear of the unknown silently torments her.

Take the time to include your wife in the decisions. Ask her what she thinks. Bring her with you to talk with your doctors. Take her to the hospital for preoperative testing. Ask her to get on the phone when your doctor calls to talk. Give her an opportunity to ask questions. Let her know that her input is important and listen to what she has to say.

Women usually do well in times of crisis, so she may serve as the steady pillar for the family during your illness. Or she may function as your 24-hour nurse when problems develop at home.

Think about this for a minute, and then take the time to include your wife in decisions. Ask her what she thinks—what sounds good, what scares her. Bring her with you to talk with your doctors. Take her to the hospital for preoperative testing. Ask her to get on the phone when your doctor calls to talk. Give her an opportunity to ask questions. Let her know that her input is important and listen to what she has to say. In these situations, women tend to have more common sense and a better ability to step back and look at the total picture.

Prostate cancer is a very personal disease. From the moment your cancer is identified until it is either cured or controlled, it is essential that you include your wife. Share your feelings with her. Openly discuss your fears and concerns with her about how this might affect your sexual relationship. You may find that this issue is less important to her than making you well and extending your life. I am always happy to see my patients bring their wives or companions with them to their appointments.

What if my wife doesn't want to be involved?
Some wives don't feel it is their place to participate in the discussions and decision making regarding their husband's care. All we can do is try to include her. Even if she won't participate in the discussion, she should be encouraged to at least listen so she can better understand what is happening to you.

I remember once I was in the middle of discussing treatment options with a patient and his wife. The gentleman stood up and interrupted our discussion to declare that if there was a chance he might lose erections, he would just rather die. His wife calmly looked over and reminded him that although their occasional sexual relations were nice, she would much rather have him around several more years than be a lonely widow simply because of an occasional lost erection. He stopped, thought about this and then asked me to continue talking about the options. As it turned out, he opted for surgery and had excellent pathology results. He did eventually regain the ability to have erections.

What if I don't agree with her opinion?

This happens occasionally. Ultimately, your course of action is your decision, to be made with your wife's input and suggestions. Try to talk about each other's feelings and thoughts. What concerns one might be of minor concern to another. Through open communication you should come to a mutual agreement. Include her in your research gathering so you can both understand the facts that are relevant to your situation.

WHAT TO TELL FAMILY
AND FRIENDS

17

The decision to tell your family, friends and neighbors about your cancer depends on your relationship with them.

I have words of caution about human nature and cancer. For reasons no one really understands, whenever the word gets out that you've been diagnosed with prostate cancer, anyone who has had prostate cancer or knows of someone with cancer will seek you out to tell you their horror stories.

Even if it's not prostate cancer, they still feel it is their responsibility to tell you how miserable Aunt Nellie was after she had radiation for breast cancer 35 years ago, or how many problems Cousin George had with his prostate cancer. I have very strong opinions about these friendly bits of advice. I have witnessed the damage they can do to my own patients' morale. I strongly encourage you to consider some things about you and your situation before heeding the advice of friends and family.

Treatments for any disease in the past have nothing to do with treatments today. Even radical prostatectomy, which is surgery to remove the cancerous prostate gland and surrounding tissues, has been much improved. The operation men are having today has significantly better results and is much better tolerated than the same operation seven years ago. Recently, a patient

Should I tell my colleagues at work about my prostate cancer?

This depends on your relationship with your co-workers and your position at work. Unfortunately, there are still many misconceptions about all forms of cancer. Telling your co-workers will definitely have some effect. It could potentially jeopardize a contract, a promotion or your day-to-day working relationships because of people's fears and confusion.

On the other hand, sharing such personal information could help you identify others who have been through similar experiences. It could also make your co-workers aware of the importance of early detection for themselves. Only you can decide if it is best to discuss your cancer with co-workers.

who had a radical prostatectomy was discharged after only 48 hours in the hospital. A few years ago that same patient would have just been getting out of the intensive care unit, with another seven to ten days of hospitalization ahead of him.

Several of my best friends were treated for cancer with good results. Why shouldn't I do what they did?

Every cancer is different, every person is unique and each patient will respond differently to each treatment. Whatever worked for someone else probably won't have relevance in your case.

I continue to hear from patients who decided on a particular treatment because of the experience of someone they know. Sometimes it was even for a different cancer, in a different area of the body, a long time ago. All I ask my patients to do is to delay making decisions until we talk and discuss all of the options and risks specific to them. Don't let preconceived notions based on hearsay and the experience of others prevent you from making the right decision for you.

Even when talking specifically about prostate cancer, several themes keep coming up when talking with others who have had treatment. Most often the stage of the cancer is different, so Cousin George's cancer may have been more or less advanced. Even if the cancers were exactly the same stage and grade, one must also consider the health, age, family history and other social and medical factors that may make your best option for treatment different.

Everyone responds to treatments differently. The best thing you can do when talking to others is take everything they say with a grain of salt, smile, thank them for their concern and file away the information. If it concerns you, then ask your urologist about what you heard and discuss whether it is a valid concern for you.

Should I tell my family?

When the time is right, yes. All male relatives are at risk and they have a need to know about your disease so that they can begin getting regular PSA tests and digital rectal exams. Those who need to know include sons, nephews, brothers, uncles and cousins. The closer the relative, the more the potential risks. Many will ignore the potential risks, while others may choose to make important dietary changes to reduce potential risks. Be sure to reassure your family that you are taking an active role in your care. Watch out for well-meaning family who want to decide what's best for you or who you should see. Their love and concern sometimes becomes a control game. Thank them for their concern and let them know you will definitely consider their input.

ACTIVE SURVEILLANCE 18

I n selected men, when the side effects of any treatments are more danger-ous than the risks of the cancer, the option of no treatment may be best. This is ideal for elderly men or men with significant health risks who have a cancer that is believed not to be significant.

Though this appears to be the safest treatment initially, there are actually a number of potentially significant risks when you choose to just observe the cancer. Observation, also called *active surveillance, watchful waiting, expectant management* or *deferred therapy*, is a reasonable option for many men in se-lected situations as long as each understands exactly what he is choosing to do. Observation does not mean we are going to forget about the cancer and hope nothing happens. Rather, this is an active program of regularly moni-toring the cancer.

I have had a number of patients who *incorrectly* believed that because they opted for watchful waiting, they could just go home and never return for follow-up exams or PSA blood tests. But this is not without potentially seri-ous risks. In the right patients, observation may very well be the best option. For others, it can be quite dangerous and short-sighted.

I have had a number of patients who incorrectly believed that because they opted for watchful waiting, they could just go home and never return for follow-up exams or PSA blood tests.

What exactly does observation mean?
Observation means to choose no active treatment for the cancer.

Why would I choose to do nothing?
When you choose this option, you and your doctors are agreeing, in essence, that you will probably die of something else before the prostate cancer can grow and cause problems or kill you. This obviously depends on a number of factors including your age, your general health, your family longevity and a little luck. This treatment is best for older men if the cancer is a low-grade, small-volume disease. It is these little cancers that are the least aggressive and the slowest growing.

Is there a problem with observation and active surveillance?
The concern with this strategy is that we know that we frequently under-estimate the grade and volume of cancer. In other words, there are times when we think the cancer is small and of little threat, when in reality it is larger and more aggressive. If you select observation based on incorrect assumptions and limited or inaccurate information, there is a good chance that if you live long enough, you will have to deal with an advanced and rapidly growing cancer. Our best diagnostic tests are still not good enough to provide an accurate picture of the cancer and the potential threat.

Everything I have read says prostate cancer is best watched with no treatment. Is this true?
There has been quite a lot of media attention regarding this philosophy, suggesting that prostate cancer is benign and will not hurt you and for many is best left untreated. Although there is some truth to this for some patients, it unfortunately will doom many young men to an unnecessarily early death.

We know that many men have prostate cancer and are never affected during their lifetime. Most men don't even know they have prostate cancer. But it is believed by urologists who specialize in prostate cancer that if we detect prostate cancer because of an abnormality on exam or because the PSA level is elevated, there is most likely a significant cancer present.

If you live long enough, and if it is allowed to grow unchecked, the cancer may very well cause symptoms. It could even result in death. Even if it is slow growing, it will gradually reach that unknown volume when it starts to grow rapidly and spread. This has been confirmed by a number of studies.

What are the chances I might die of prostate cancer if I choose to do nothing?

Assuming you do not have advanced or aggressive disease, 15% or more of men who think they have a small, insignificant cancer and do nothing will eventually develop advanced prostate cancer and die from it within the first ten years. If you live longer than ten years, the chances for rapid growth and spread of the cancer and death go up dramatically. The majority of men who

Who is a good candidate for "active surveillance"?

The ideal person for simple observation is an elderly man in his late 70s or 80s, ill with a limited long-term life expectancy. Likewise, men in their 60s and early 70s with other potentially life-threatening health problems should probably avoid treatment. The key is that the treatment should never be worse than the disease.

The answer to the question "What's going to get you first?" is simply a guess, an odds game. On one extreme, you want to avoid unnecessary treatment and potential risks. At the other end, it is always sad when someone chooses a conservative approach only to die later from a treatable prostate cancer. This sometimes happens either because they lived longer than they had anticipated or because the cancer was more significant than they had assumed. If you live long enough, an untreated cancer may very well kill you.

live long enough will die as a result of the cancer between 14 and 17 years after diagnosis.

What factors should encourage me to choose active surveillance?
Observation may be a reasonable choice if:
- You have less than five years of life expectancy.
- The cancer is low grade and well differentiated.
- You have low PSA levels.

On rare occasions I have found a tiny amount of cancer at a TURP (prostate resection) and recommended simple monitoring of PSA levels. If you are in your 70s or 80s and generally quite ill with a number of other health problems, then the cancer can be a higher grade or stage, and observation may still be a good choice. In this situation, the treatment may actually be worse than the disease.

Who should not choose surveillance?
Again, it depends on the specifics of the cancer and your health. If you think you will not live long enough for the untreated cancer to cause a problem, then opt for observation. But if you are young (early 70s or less), healthy and will most likely live for several years, then it would be in your best interest to choose some form of treatment. If left to grow long enough, even many small cancers can become potentially dangerous, spread and kill.

But what if my cancer is one of those that really is not significant?
Then you don't need any treatment. But be forewarned: It is difficult to determine with certainty if you are the rare man with a prostate cancer that doesn't need any treatment at all. Most often, a cancer is large enough to warrant some kind of treatment. If it was discovered, chances are it is significant.

How will my progress be monitored?
You will need to have the PSA blood test on a regular basis. In addition, you should have periodic prostate exams, plus urinalysis to check for blood and a brief review of symptoms or concerns.

How frequently do I need to be monitored?

This depends on how concerned you and your doctor are about progression of the cancer. It is probably reasonable to check the PSA every four to six months. The longer you have a stable PSA, usually the longer you can wait between intervals of each PSA check. This is something you will decide with your doctor.

Why can't I check the PSA level more often so we can tell if the cancer starts to grow?

If you check a PSA too often, such as every month or two, you may end up getting excited over some minor but usual fluctuation from test to test.

While I am in active surveillance, do I need a repeat prostate ultrasound or biopsy?

No. We know you have cancer and it won't just fade away. But we are hoping it will remain small and slow growing. Having additional biopsies won't add any significant new information.

Should I get a repeat bone scan?

Only if the PSA level begins to climb rapidly, suggesting fast growth. Otherwise, the PSA and exam should be adequate to monitor the cancer and be sure it is not growing.

What about those news reports saying most men with prostate cancer will not die of it?

This is a true but somewhat misleading statement. Autopsy studies on men who died of other causes have shown that a large part of the aging male population will have prostate cancer at the time of their death and not even know it. But this includes even tiny specks of low-grade disease, as well as those with large volumes of cancer and metastatic disease.

More important is what happens to those men who are diagnosed with a significant cancer, as determined by the PSA, exam, biopsies and ultrasound findings. If these men live long enough, the cancer will continue to grow unchecked and ultimately can spread. If there is a significant cancer but you

Several years ago I had the great pleasure of getting to know Matthew, a distinguished political person with a zeal for life. After a complete workup, I diagnosed his prostate cancer. Matthew is a young man, 62, in the prime of his life, but he also has significant heart disease. Because of this, he strongly believes that it is best to just monitor his prostate cancer rather than take all the risks and possibly suffer the side effects of either surgery or radiation. He wants to maximize the quality of his life for as long as he can. I am very happy to participate in his care on these terms.

are older with only a few years to live, and if you are in poor health, then it is reasonable to opt for no treatment and just monitoring of the PSA.

Another factor we have to consider is how fast the cancer is growing. We call this *doubling time.* This tells us how long it takes for a set amount of cancer to double in size. Fortunately for many men, this is so slow that the cancers are seldom detected and the men live a full life, never being diagnosed or treated for prostate cancer. Because this represents the majority of men, it skews the statistics and that results in confusion. It is generally accepted that if we find a cancer, it is significant and should be treated. If it has a fast-doubling time of one year or less, that suggests a fast-growing cancer.

What if I want treatment but my primary-care doctor and my urologist both want me to pursue watchful waiting?

This usually means your doctors are worried that the treatments are potentially more threatening to your health than the disease. I have had a patient with multiple serious health problems who wanted a radical prostatectomy. I was able to persuade him to consider other options, and he finally consented to have radiation. As expected, he did well with the radiation, although he continued to have problems with his heart and even had a series of strokes.

If your doctor and urologist are trying to talk you out of an aggressive treatment, then you should listen to what they are saying. If you don't understand why they are trying to persuade you to avoid therapy, ask them!

What if my primary-care doctor and my urologist both want me to
have surgery or radiation but I want active surveillance?
This question is just the opposite of the preceding one. Here, your doctors believe that the cancer is significant enough to be a threat to your life and that it is worth worth taking whatever risks are involved to address it. This might be based on the PSA, the biopsy results, your age or your general health. You may think you're old with a limited life span, when you actually are in great shape and may live a lot longer than you realize. If you are the only one leaning toward observation, I would suggest you reevaluate and perhaps seek additional opinions.

What if my primary-care doctor says I shouldn't do anything, but my
urologist is recommending aggressive surgery or radiation?
This is a potentially sticky situation with no clear answer. It's difficult to know what each physician's opinions and recommendations are based on.

In my experience, this conflicting advice most often occurs because the primary-care doctor doesn't understand the potential seriousness of the cancer or the limited risks of therapy. Many doctors believe the surgery or radiation is far worse than it really is. Most often, the primary-care doctor has been influenced by the news reports that suggest prostate cancer is a benign disease. Primary-care doctors may even consider the urologist's advice as self-serving or inappropriate.

Occasionally, I hear of a urologist who recommends that an elderly patient with serious health problems undergo surgical removal of the prostate or radiation therapy—the patient's life span is quite limited. I'm not sure who or what that urologist is treating. This is a situation where a second opinion can help clear up the confusion.

Whenever there is confusion or conflicting advice, I advise patients to seek an additional opinion from a urologist who deals with a large number of prostate-cancer patients.

If the cancer appears to be growing during surveillance, would I then
need to have treatment?
This is the reason for this category—to keep an eye on the tumor, and if there are signs of significant growth, then to treat it accordingly. The treatment

? *While I'm under observation, how will we know if there is continued growth of the cancer?*

Usually there will be a regular trend of increasing PSA levels over time. I prefer to have two or three PSA checks done annually to watch out for an elevation that is not just lab fluctuation. Sometimes the exam can change with a nodule becoming larger or harder.

selected depends on how fast the cancer appears to be growing and your general health. If I become worried that the cancer is starting to act more aggressively, and if I am concerned that the growth may cause problems or ultimately kill you, then I would recommend the start of treatment. This is why active surveillance is sometimes called *deferred therapy*. We will wait and see if the cancer may be a threat to you.

If I choose active surveillance, at what point would treatment be started if the cancer does start to grow?

There is no exact answer to this question. A persistent elevation, with each PSA being higher and higher over time, worries me. If the PSA and exam suggest cancer is growing, then I would recommend you start a treatment that is appropriate for the specifics of the cancer, your age and your health.

At what point is it clear that something needs to be done and that observation is not effective?

The big question (and at the same time the big problem) with active surveillance is: What is the end point we are waiting for? At what point do we agree that, despite our hopes that the cancer is insignificant, it appears there are real changes that suggest tumor progression?

Is this end point a change in the digital exam or perhaps an increase in PSA levels? How much of a PSA elevation makes us worried? At what point along the course of elevation do we admit that observation is no longer appropriate and consider options for treatment? Do we wait, as some suggest, until symptoms develop?

My preference would be to agree that a continually elevating PSA is consistent with tumor growth, assuming there is no urinary-tract infection, and early treatment will hopefully result in better long-term results. That is when I would want to start treatment.

If we watch the situation and at some point there is evidence of cancer growth, will the options be different from those that existed when the cancer was first diagnosed?

We hope not. We would like to think that in the ideal situation, a healthy male who is on the borderline between treatment and watchful waiting will not go beyond the curable phase if he chooses to wait until there is early evidence of cancer progression.

However, recent studies show the best time to treat many prostate cancers is when the PSA level is 4.0 or less. If we wait until the PSA is greater than 10.0, for example, the odds that the cancer has started to spread through the wall of the prostate go up dramatically.

For many men, the treatment choices would be the same, although the odds of being successful in removing or treating all the cancer may be less.

Could the cancer actually go to the lymph nodes or the bones while it is being watched closely?

This is always a possibility. We have no way to know for sure that the cancer remaining is confined to the prostate gland. The PSA check is only a very rough estimate. The problem with waiting until there are definite signs of growth before you start treatment is that we may wait too long. Whether or not we pass that critical point when the cancer starts to spread varies from person to person. It is always possible that the cancer will spread to the surrounding tissues or to the lymph nodes or bones during this time.

If left untreated and the cancer continues to grow, how long until it causes problems?

If we had the answer, we would know who should and who shouldn't be treated and which treatment is best. This uncertainty is the dilemma of prostate cancer. Many men will not live long enough for the cancer to be a threat to them, while others may have rapid growth or live long enough to have problems because of the cancer.

Recent long-term studies show that if you live ten years or more after diagnosis of cancer, and you have not had any treatment, your odds of dying from prostate cancer begin to increase dramatically. Even if you live only a few years and have chosen to do nothing, the cancer may cause problems. The cancer may grow, spread and require some treatment, possibly years before the ten-year point.

In general, if you have just a few years of expected survival, and the cancer is not advanced, you may want to at least consider active surveillance.

RADIATION—EXTERNAL-BEAM/IMRT THERAPY

19

R adiation therapy is a well-established technique of killing cancer cells with one of two different types of radiation that are used to treat prostate cancer today. According to Dr. David Beyer of Scottsdale, Arizona, who is one of the world's leading prostate cancer radiation therapists, the most effective of external-beam therapies are *3-D conformal* and *IMRT (intensity modulated radiation therapy)*. These are now considered the gold standard of radiation techniques.

There is also *interstitial radiotherapy*, in which radioactive pellets are placed within the prostate. This technique, also known as *radioactive seed therapy* or *brachytherapy*, is discussed in Chapter 20.

How does radiation work without hurting normal tissues?
Most malignant cells are less efficient in repairing the injury from radiation than normal cells are. Therefore, most malignant tumors can be destroyed by amounts of radiation that don't hurt normal tissues. There will be some normal cells that will die, but the body can repair this damage with normal cell growth and replacement.

	External-Beam	Radioactive Seeds
Treatment Time	7 weeks	1–2 days
Anesthesia	No	Yes
Hospitalization	No	Yes
Fatigue	Yes	No
Pain	Not Usually	Temporary
Bleeding	Possible, Delayed	Infrequent
Incontinence	Infrequent	Infrequent
Impotence	25%–50%	25%–60%
Bladder/Rectal Irritation	10%–15%	10%–15%
Severe Reaction (Bleeding, Fistula, Pain)	1%	1%
Long-Term Effectiveness	Good, Recurrences 7–10 years	Good for selected patients

Comparison of external-beam radiation versus radioactive seeds

What is external-beam radiation therapy (EBRT)?
This is the term for a specific radiation technique used to treat many types of cancers in the body. Beams of high-energy radiation are focused from outside the body (hence *external-beam*) onto the target area.

What are the types of external-beam radiation?
The two main categories of radiation are 3-D conformal and IMRT.

What is 3-D conformal radiation therapy?
This is a widely used improvement in standard external-beam therapy where computer-generated CT-scan images and a fitted brace are used to focus the radiation beams more precisely. This techinique is believed to be more accurate in focusing the radiation to the prostate. It allows higher doses of radiation to the prostate with reduced doses to the surrounding tissues and the

very sensitive rectal wall. There are fewer side effects with 3-D conformal therapy than the old, external-beam techniques.

What exactly is IMRT?

IMRT stands for *intensity modulated radiation therapy*. This new technique is not just an improvement, but rather an entirely new idea in radiation therapy. IMRT uses a highly focused, computer-directed, pencil-sized micro-beams of radiation that are precisely matched to the shape of the prostate and tumor. This results in minimal damage to surrounding tissues with a maximum dose of killing radiation to the target area. IMRT is felt to offer fewer side effects and better results. Recent studies have shown excellent results using IMRT after nerve-sparing prostatectomy for those men at high risk for return of the cancer.

Can radiation hurt me?

In uncontrolled amounts, radiation can be quite dangerous and even deadly. But radiation therapists use information from your CT scans and knowledge about your particular cancer and anatomy to custom-design a pattern and dose of radiation. This approach maximizes the killing of cancer cells in the target area with minimal damage to adjacent normal tissues. This specificity is why everything is so precisely calculated.

How should I decide if radiation therapy is best for me?

You will need to consult with a radiation therapist, who is a physician trained and experienced in treating cancer with radiation. At that time you will review the important facts regarding your situation to decide if you are a candidate for radiation. You will also discuss potential risks and side effects, as well as the possible benefits.

What happens to me if I choose external-beam therapy?

You will have what's called a *simulation*, where special X-rays are taken to help determine the dose and focus the radiation. Shortly thereafter, you will start your treatments based on a set schedule, usually at the same time every day, until completed.

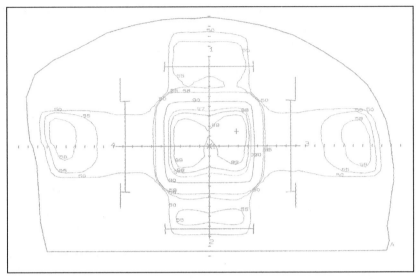

SIMULATION FOR EXTERNAL-BEAM RADIATION. Computerized drawing
of prostate from different angles, showing exact dose of radiation that will be given
to the prostate and surrounding tissues in subsequent radiation therapy.

How quickly could I start radiation treatments?

When you have decided to proceed with radiation, you should be able to
have a simulation and start treatment within a few days, depending on the
facility and the doctor. Most often your treatments will begin within a few
weeks. There is usually no real urgency to start immediately. Chances are
you have had this cancer for many years and probably decades.

What is the length of treatment?

The full course of standard external-beam therapy takes about six and one-
half to seven weeks, Monday through Friday. It was always felt that with the
radiation techniques and the nature of cancer-cell growth, the time it takes
to complete the radiation cannot be shortened. Because of its more precise
nature, IMRT takes eight to nine weeks to complete.

New studies are looking at a much quicker treatment course, called *dose
fractionation schemes*. Early experimental trials suggest that in the future, if
long-term results are good, the entire course could be completed in five
weeks. One study is looking at effectiveness of giving all the radiation in just

one week. The big concern is long-term survival and side effects from much higher doses.

How much time does the radiation treatment take every day?

Radiation takes just ten to fifteen minutes each day. There is time to set up and get you back out and home or back to work.

Why is it given only Monday through Friday?

This schedule allows normal body cells to recover during the brief time off each weekend. This results in better killing of cancer cells gradually over time.

Who actually does the radiation treatments?

Radiation therapists who are specially trained to treat cancers perform treatments. These physicians have completed a residency of several years in radiation therapy for cancer treatment. The doctors work closely with physicists, radiation-therapy technicians and radiation nurses to determine exactly how to treat and monitor you throughout and after the therapy.

Do all radiation doctors get the same results?

Much depends on you, your anatomy and the cancer. Just as important is the skill and expertise of your radiation team. There are some doctors who focus their practices on prostate cancer and so would be expected to get better results with fewer complications.

Does radiation kill the cancer cells?

The main goal of radiation treatment is to control cancer growth and prevent the spread of cancer. There continues to be debate as to whether radiation kills the cancer cells or simply stuns them. It really doesn't make any difference as long as you live a normal life span without signs or symptoms of the cancer.

What are the advantages of radiation therapy?

Radiation offers good treatment for the right candidate without the standard risks that go along with surgery and anesthesia. There is no risk of surgical

EXTERNAL-BEAM RADIATION THERAPY

Advantages	*Disadvantages*
No surgery, no anesthesia	No lymph-node or prostate analysis
No transfusion risk	Possible irritation of bladder and/or
Less impotence than surgery	rectum (10%–15%)
Incontinence unlikely (less than 5%)	Rare risk of serious complications
Good control of cancer	(1%)
	Monday through Friday for 7 weeks
	Possible local return of cancer in
	7–10 years

bleeding, no hospitalization, usually no pain, no heart attacks, strokes or blood clots. I believe radiation is a very effective conservative approach.

It is ideal for the man who cannot or will not have his prostate removed, or whose age or health makes his surgery risks higher than those for other men. Radiation provides survival results equal to surgery for a man with a life expectancy of about seven to ten years.

What kind of rectal problems can occur?
There is a risk of radiation injury of the rectum or rectal wall, called *radiation proctitis*, which can result in irritative symptoms including pain, changed frequency of bowel movements, and urgency to have bowel movements. It can also result in bleeding, chronic burning and rectal discharge or leakage. If you already have significant rectal or bowel problems, you should avoid external-beam radiation, because this therapy will usually make your symptoms much worse.

What can be done to treat diarrhea and stomach upset?
Most often these symptoms are only mild to moderate and will go away on their own. Occasionally the radiation doses or frequency of treatments must be temporarily reduced until your symptoms start to go away. Certain medications often can be given to reduce your symptoms.

> *What are the main side effects of radiation?*
>
> The most common side effect is fatigue in some men, which appears toward the end of treatment. There also is about a 10% to 15% risk of developing some degree of bladder and/or rectal irritation. Irritation to the bladder can cause symptoms similar to a bladder infection, such as burning with urination and the sense of urgency to urinate.
>
> Sometimes blood in the urine can be seen after radiation. This bleeding can occur at any time after the treatment is over, even many years later. However, it is very important not to assume that any blood in the urine is a consequence of prior radiation. A complete evaluation by a urologist is necessary if blood is seen to be sure you do not have a bladder tumor.
>
> Some patients also experience frequent bowel movements, diarrhea and/or stomach problems.
>
> There is a 30% to 50% risk of developing problems with erections, including total impotence, because of radiation damage to small blood vessels and the nerves responsible for erections. There is less than a 5% risk of urinary leakage, a potentially serious side effect.

What can be done to treat bladder irritation?

Sometimes your doctor will prescribe medications to help to relax the bladder and make it less irritable. These include Detrol LA, Ditropan XL, Sanctura XR, VESicare, Urispas and Pyridium for burning on urination.

Are these side effects permanent?

These side effects, if they occur, usually go away with completion of the radiation treatments. Although it is uncommon, some men complain of continued problems with urinating, with bowel movements or with lingering fatigue.

What about hair loss with radiation?

Hair loss occurs only in the area that is receiving the largest dose of radiation. Radiation of the prostate does not cause hair on your head to fall out. You

Is there a problem with nausea during radiation?

Nausea is associated with radiation to the abdomen or chest, where the intestines and stomach might be radiated. With radiation of the prostate, because of its location, nausea is almost unheard of as a side effect.

might see some changes in the hair on your lower abdomen or pubic area, but that's about it.

Does radiation therapy hurt?
No, there is no pain associated with the radiation therapy itself. The exception would be if the radiation irritates the bladder or rectum.

Does radiation burn the skin?
No. Modern radiation techniques do not result in skin damage that was common with radiation treatments decades ago.

Does it make a difference how soon radiation is begun?
As long as treatment begins within a reasonable time after the cancer is diagnosed, there should be no serious problems. A delay of a month or two or even a little more shouldn't affect long-term results in most men. Your long-term results depend more on your particular situation, plus the grade and stage of the cancer. I usually counsel my patients to proceed relatively soon with the treatment, just to be sure.

What are the disadvantages of radiation therapy?
The length of treatment—nearly two months or more—can be a real nuisance and inconvenience for many men. If you live close to a radiation-treatment facility, then it may be convenient. Unfortunately, some men may live a long distance from a treatment facility. Most men can't move near a facility for two months. Few have the financial resources to take off extended time from work.

Another disadvantage of radiation is that it offers no opportunity to evaluate the lymph nodes or prostate to be sure the treatment is indeed the correct one.

Perhaps the most controversial disadvantage is that radiation therapy is believed by many experts to be not as effective as radical surgery for patients who may have a life expectancy longer than seven to ten years. Others disagree and feel it may be equally effective for many men.

What are the long-term results of radiation therapy?

Most experts will agree that radiation therapy is as effective as radical prostatectomy for the first seven to ten years after treatment. There is some debate about long-term treatment results. For correctly selected men, radiation can provide excellent long-term, cancer-free and survival results.

Will radiation therapy cure me?

The goal of radiation treatment is to kill cancer cells. Studies show that sometimes the cancer can still be present but inactive, or dormant, even years after treatment. The presence of cancer shouldn't be a problem as long as it stays inactive. This is why you always need to be regularly monitored with the PSA blood test following radiation. Then, if the PSA level starts to go up (called *biochemical recurrence*), suggesting that cancer is growing again, the doctors can get a better idea of how fast it is growing and if there's any reason for concern. It may grow so slowly after radiation that it will never be a problem to you during your lifetime. Some doctors believe the radiation may not cure you, but it may stun the cancer and render it inactive.

How does radiation cause urine leakage, or incontinence?

Radiation can cause scarring and injury to the muscle fibers located at the bladder neck or at the sphincter. This is usually a slow process, and for most men it is relatively uncommon.

When these tissues are damaged, they can no longer snug up tightly. Also, the muscles of the bladder neck can't squeeze effectively at the sphincter. This means that some urine may leak out. Leakage is most commonly associated with coughing, sneezing or straining. Some men are aware of leakage only when they stand up, run or move around. Although this leakage is usually permanent, most men don't regard it as a significant problem.

Can radiation cause erectile dysfunction?
Yes. One-third to one-half of men treated by radiation may experience some degree of decreased erections. This problem may take a year or more to manifest itself, but impotence is a real problem that cannot be avoided for some men. Radiation may cause decreased erections by damaging the small blood vessels and nerves that are necessary for erections.

Will radiation affect my desire for sex?
Radiation does not impact on a man's sex drive. As the treatments go on, fatigue could affect your desire for sexual relations. Some men are reluctant to have sex during treatments because of fears regarding the cancer. Truthfully, there is no medical reason to abstain from having sex.

Over time, for some men, the ability to have an erection may decrease or even go away totally. This is not usually associated with a lack of interest, but is a physical problem.

How soon can I go back to work?
If you are one of the few who develops some lasting fatigue, you may need to take a few weeks or more off until your strength returns. One of the advantages of radiation treatment is that many men can continue to work or participate in activities such as golf, hiking, swimming or tennis during and after the treatments. Some patients find that a daily nap enables them to carry on their normal routine.

Do I need repeat biopsies after radiation?
No. The results of a repeat biopsy would not affect how I would care for my patient, so I don't see any need to put him through an uncomfortable and unnecessary test. Now that I've said that, there will always be special situations that may require biopsies.

What kind of follow-up will happen after my radiation treatment?
It is best to be followed regularly with PSA tests and prostate exams.

What can be expected to happen to the PSA level after radiation?
With ideal prostate cancer-cell death or injury from the radiation, the PSA level should drop, ideally below 0.5, over a period of several months.

> **Options if PSA Increases After Radiation**
> - Repeat PSA in 3 to 4 months
> - Possible bone scan
> - Hormone therapy for presumed recurrent/metastatic disease
> - Salvage prostatectomy—high risk
> - Cryotherapy/HIFU

What if the PSA level doesn't drop after radiation?
This usually means that there are cancer cells elsewhere in the body that were not affected by radiation. Occasionally some men will have a temporary rise (PSA bounce) in PSA before it drops back down again.

Is radiation therapy a good treatment for aggressive high-grade cancers?
No. Radiation therapy is less effective with large or aggressive cancers. It should still be considered as a treatment option, because surgery and hormone therapy are also less effective with this type of cancer. The nice point about radiation is that it can be safely added on after surgery, if needed.

Can I do anything to get better results if I have a high-grade cancer and decide to have radiation therapy?
For many men who are at high risk because of a high-grade, aggressive cancer (Gleason 8 to 10) or one that the doctors feel may be starting to grow outside the prostate (Stage C/T3), eliminating the male hormones (via hormone therapy) prior to and during radiation therapy actually provides better long-term results. Studies now suggest that pretreatment with hormone-blocking medications makes the radiation more effective. Some chemotherapy medications actually makes the cancer cells more sensitive to the lethal effects of radiation.

Can radiation actually stimulate the cancer's growth?
No, but it can sometimes appear to do so. If there is cancer outside the field of radiation, it would continue to grow and lead to problems or even death.

> *Will there be any problems if I want to take a break halfway*
> *through radiation treatments?*
>
> **?**
>
> Yes. This could seriously reduce the effectiveness of the
> radiation treatments. Again, they are calculated to provide the
> maximum killing dose and to reach all the cancer cells in
> critical phases of growth during the treatment time. If you stop
> midtreatment for a while, you may end up with worse long-
> term results. It is advisable to plan your schedule so you can
> complete treatments as prescribed by the radiation therapist.

Will the large size of my prostate influence how well the radiation will work?

Yes. Radiation works less effectively for very large prostates. This is why you need to discuss this option with your radiation therapist to see if this is a good option for you.

Should I have surgery to make the prostate smaller?

No. Surgery simply to reduce the prostate size before radiation is not very effective and will often increase the potential complications. In addition, you would be taking on additional and unnecessary risks of surgery and anesthesia.

If I get hormone therapy or chemotherapy before radiation, should I stay on it afterward?

For patients with an aggressive cancer, this may be a good idea. Some studies suggest this may be very effective, when compared with radiation alone. This combination is ideal for the patient for whom radiation by itself will most likely fail to control the cancer.

If I have difficulty urinating, will radiation make it worse?

It can. There is usually some initial swelling of the prostate with radiation treatment. If the enlargement is already causing problems, then radiation can actually make it worse before it gets better. Often the use of alpha-blockers helps to reduce these symptoms.

Does it make a difference if my doctor wants me to have a TURP,
instead of a biopsy, to look for cancer?

If you have problems urinating and potentially have cancer, do the biopsy first. If it comes back showing cancer, then you might want to have your prostate totally removed and solve the blockage problem. If the biopsies are all normal, then you can address the blockage with your doctors, again starting with medications such as alpha-blockers. A TURP before radiation increases your risks for complications.

Are there any very serious complications with radiation?

There is a 1% chance that radiation may result in severe pain or bleeding, or the development of an abnormal connection between the bladder and rectum, called a *fistula*. If a fistula develops, it requires surgery for urine drainage to a bag (called a *urostomy*) and/or for intestinal drainage to a bag (called a *colostomy*). The more experienced your radiation therapist, the less likely you will have a serious problem.

Can I have radiation if I am taking Coumadin blood thinner?

Yes, although you will need to discuss this with your doctors. Delayed bleeding from the bladder is one potential side effect that may not happen for up to a few years after radiation. If your doctor tells you not to stop taking Coumadin for any reason, then you should probably not have radiation. This is a point on which experts do not agree. If you are considering radiation and you take Coumadin, talk about your concerns with your radiation therapist.

How long after radiation can I expect to see blood in my urine?

This can occur right away but is most common a year or more after treatments are over. The blood can be just little clots, it can show up as a discoloration of urine or it can be quite severe and heavy. If it is a problem, talk to your doctors right away.

Why is there bleeding after the radiation is over?

Bleeding is from radiation damage to the normal tissues and blood vessels that line the inside of the bladder and prostate. The radiation makes the blood vessels very fragile and easily broken. Sometimes the bleeding starts after straining to have a bowel movement or after sex. Sometimes bleeding starts for no reason.

How is the bleeding treated?

If the bleeding is severe and heavy, first your doctors need to evaluate where the bleeding is coming from. Although it is common to see blood in the urine after radiation, blood can also come from a bladder cancer, kidney tumor, kidney stone or a number of other problems. Sometimes you may need to have a kidney X-ray such as a CT scan to look at the kidneys, ureters and bladder. You almost always will need a cystoscopy to look at the bladder lining and possibly biopsies of any suspicious areas. If the bleeding is severe, the urologist may want to cauterize (burn with electricity or laser) the bleeding spots, usually under anesthesia. Because the bleeding most often will stop on its own, the most common way to treat minor bleeding is with time and increased fluids.

What if it continues to bleed?

Other treatment choices include rinsing a solution of alum through a catheter into the bladder. This solution uses the same substance as a styptic pencil that stops bleeding on your face after shaving. Some doctors put a formaldehyde solution into the bladder under anesthesia to chemically seal all blood vessels.

Some studies have shown that briefly putting the patient inside a hyperbaric oxygen tank every day for a month can also reduce and prevent future bleeding. Unfortunately, these special oxygen devices are usually found only in large medical centers. Hyperbaric oxygen is increased oxygen under pressure, as used for deep-sea divers suffering from the bends.

There are also some medications that may help to stop bleeding or stabilize the delicate blood vessel walls. One medication, Amicar, can be given as a pill or put directly into the bladder to stop bleeding.

For severe bleeding the radiologist can place a tiny coil and block off blood vessels that are bleeding. In rare cases, an incision may be needed under anesthesia for the surgeon to identify and tie off arteries that take blood to the bladder. Even more dramatic would be the removal of the bladder entirely, though this is extremely rare.

TREATMENT FOR BLEEDING AFTER RADIATION

Do nothing
Cauterize
Alum irrigations into bladder
Amicar—bladder irrigations or pills
Formaldehyde into bladder
Hyperbaric oxygen
Surgery

What is IGRT?

This is new form of IMRT with active image guidance. What this means is that the target is adjusted daily to account for minor changes in your body. The thought is that this will make IMRT even more precise with even fewer complications and side effects. There are some studies looking at doing real-time adjustments while the radiation is being given.

What about proton-beam therapy?

This technique is available only in selected centers around the United States. Very powerful beams of protons are focused onto the prostate. The idea is that high doses offer better results. Those who promote this treatment claim that it works well. The remainder of radiation therapists are still waiting to see long-term results. Costs are substantially higher than standard IMRT, which also provides high doses.

RADIATION—RADIOACTIVE SEED IMPLANTS

20

Treatment with radioactive seeds has become standard over the past 15 years. With new improvements in techniques and equipment, seed therapy results are even better than before. Called *interstitial radiotherapy*, or *brachytherapy*, these improved methods offer the promise of a quick, minimally invasive treatment option, with good control in men with cancer confined to the prostate.

The "seeds" are actually tiny rice-sized pellets specially treated to be radioactive. Each seed gives off a known amount of radioactivity into surrounding tissues.

Dr. David Beyer, one of the leading experts in brachytherapy, notes that when these seeds are permanently placed inside the prostate gland, the very high dose of radioactivity from the seeds will kill the adjacent cancer cells without the problems and lengthy treatment time that can be seen with external-beam radiation.

Originally, *gold* or *iodine* seeds were placed surgically, but men continued to have problems with the return and spread of cancer. Newer seeds were developed, including *iodine, iridium, palladium* and more recently *cesium*. Each of these types of radioactive pellets gives off a calculated amount of radiation. With this information, radiation therapists can decide how many seeds are needed and at what dose to adequately treat a specific prostate cancer.

Why are there different types of radioactive pellets?

Each seed type has definite advantages and disadvantages with its use. For example, new trials with cesium seeds, which are the most radioactive, may offer the best ability to kill some types of cancer cells. But the very same energy level that may make them good could very well lead to increased risks for radiation irritation of the rectum or bladder. Though rare, the radiation given off from the seeds can irritate or burn sensitive tissues of the rectal wall, which lies adjacent to the prostate. In very rare cases, a colostomy may be necessary.

Why isn't everyone with prostate cancer being treated with interstitial therapy?

There are still some uncertainties regarding the long-term results. In other words, for correctly selected men, treatment with radioactive seeds appears to be equivalent to IMRT up to about seven to ten years or more. Beyond that, we don't know. This raises some concerns for younger men with a long-term expected survival. The ideal candidates for seeds are older men with small volumes of low-grade cancer, a PSA of less than 10 and small prostates.

Recent studies show that even with newer advances, the dose to the prostate can vary dramatically within the gland.

Who should not have interstitial therapy?

Men with a large, high-grade cancer, a PSA of more than 10, a Gleason sum of 7 or more or a large prostate are more likely to fail this treatment alone.

How are the seeds put in place?

Most often they are inserted through the skin of the perineum, just under the scrotum and in front of the anus. Because this procedure would otherwise be painful, it is done under anesthesia. This could be either *general* anesthesia where you are put to sleep, or a *spinal* or *epidural* anesthesia where just the area below the waist is anesthetized.

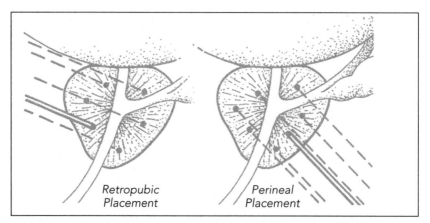

PLACEMENT OF SEEDS. Radioactive seeds are placed through hollow needles, directly into the prostate gland. Direction of implantation is more parallel to the urethra than diagrammed here.

Each seed is carefully placed in a predetermined location and depth as follows: A specially designed plastic template steers the preloaded needles into correct position. The position is confirmed with rectal ultrasound that is used to monitor the seed placement. The radioactive seeds are then inserted through these needles.

How long will I be in the hospital for placing the seeds?
Usually no longer than overnight, if that long. Most men go home that day.

How long does it take to insert radioactive seeds?
The average time to insert the seeds, including preparation and care afterward, is about one and a half to two hours.

How long am I asleep?
You will sleep for the entire time the seeds are being inserted. You first wake up from anesthesia and become aware it is all over when you are in the recovery room, or even in your hospital room.

Does it hurt to have seeds inserted?

The seeds are inserted through tiny holes in the skin under the scrotum while you are under anesthesia. If you have any pain or discomfort, it is usually described as soreness or ache in the perineal area for a week or two.

What are the main complications and side effects of seed placement?

Most often the biggest problem has to do with irritation of the urinary tract. Symptoms include an urgency to urinate with little warning, increased need to urinate frequently, possible burning or irritation with urination and blood in the urine or semen. In addition, some men can experience similar irritation of the rectum with pain, burning, frequency and urgency to have bowel movements. There is a chance of impotence. Other potential problems include prostate infections or urinary retention.

How are these symptoms treated?

Some medications can be prescribed to reduce these symptoms and soothe an irritated bladder or rectum. Alpha-blockers such as Flomax, Rapaflo or Uroxatral can improve urination symptoms. Sometimes stool softeners can help as well. Occasionally, pain medication can reduce symptoms, and even steroid enemas have been used to reduce symptoms associated with irritation.

Do the symptoms start up right away?

Not always. Some men complain of increasing symptoms of bladder and/or rectal irritation even 12 to 18 months after treatments are over.

What are my risks for leaking urine after seed implantation?

If you have had a TURP, there is more risk. However, this is usually still infrequent. (I know of many patients implanted after a TURP with a very low risk. Patients who have a TURP after seed implantation, however, have a much higher incidence of incontinence.)

What else can I expect following seed placement?

Some men complain of seeing blood in their semen, a condition called *hematospermia*. This is normal. Other uncommon problems include soreness of the testicles and, very rarely, pain with ejaculation.

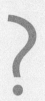

What are the odds of becoming impotent after seed placement?

This is quoted at about 25%, but it really depends more on how good an erection you are getting before any treatments. The better your erection is before treatment, the better it will probably be after treatment. The actual rate of impotence varies from 25% to 61%. As with any operator-dependent treatment, the more skilled and experienced your radiation therapist, the lower your complication rates. Choose your radiation doctor like you would a surgeon—find the one with the best skills and track record.

Will there be pain with ejaculation following placement of the seeds?

Yes, there can be. This is probably temporary irritation of surrounding tissues from the needle placement of the seeds and from inflammation caused by radioactivity. It usually passes with time.

What about evaluating the lymph nodes?

Interstitial seeds can't deliver radiation to the lymph nodes that drain the prostate. If the cancer is low-grade and the PSA level is less than 10, then it is not likely the cancer has spread. In such cases, the nodes would go without evaluation or treatment. The seed technique alone is best for those men who most likely do not have cancer in the lymph nodes.

Can I have the seeds removed if there is a problem?

No. After the seeds are inserted, they have to be left in place permanently.

Is radiation from seeds a threat to my pets, wife or friends who may be near me?

No, not at all. The dose of radiation is calculated to affect the prostate tissues immediately adjacent to the pellets. Even with this in mind, some radiation therapists suggest, just to be sure, that you not hold young babies or children in your lap or be next to them or pregnant women for an extended time after the seeds are placed. These precautions even apply to women that might become pregnant. Better to be safe than sorry.

How many seeds are placed?
This depends on the type of seeds selected and the size of the prostate gland. The number of seeds can range from 40 to 150, with the average about 80 using current techniques.

How long are the seeds radioactive?
This depends on the type of seeds selected and how much radiation needs to be delivered to the prostate. Some pellets may have a long radioactive life, but they won't be as powerful as other types that may have more energy to give off in a shorter time. In general, it is safe to say the seeds are usually radioactive for days to weeks to months.

What is the youngest age a man should be to consider radioactive seeds?
This would depend on several factors, including specifics of the cancer (grade, stage, PSA levels, exam findings, volume of disease) in addition to his age, health, longevity and access to other treatment choices.

Is seed therapy a good option if I do not live near a radiation facility for external-beam therapy and cannot or will not have surgery?
Yes, this would be a great choice in this situation.

Is there an age at which I should consider seed therapy?
If you are a candidate for IMRT, then you may also be a candidate for this technique.

Are the seeds as effective as IMRT?
In the short term, seven to ten years, the effectiveness may be as good. The true test of this option rests with long-term results, which are not yet known. Many physicians now offer both radioactive seeds and IMRT. The biggest problem with all radiation therapies is that the treatments are based

RADIOACTIVE SEEDS

Advantages	Disadvantages
25% to 61% impotence	Lymph nodes not evaluated
Quick recovery	Possible irritation of bladder and/or rectum
Short hospitalization	
No transfusions	Unknown long-term results
	Expensive

(Note: Cost for an average brachytherapy in 2009 is comparable to that of IMRT or a radical prostatectomy. Total cost could run from $15,000 to $25,000, though this is almost always covered by insurance or Medicare.)

on assumptions that the biopsy report is accurate. Usually we are right. Occasionally we are not.

Do seeds ever come out on their own in the urine or semen?
Yes, these tiny seeds can work their way out into the urethra, often in the first few days or weeks. Do *not* touch a seed with your fingers.

Can the seeds cause damage to surrounding tissues?
Hopefully not. It is always possible that radioactive pellets that lie nearby may irritate the bladder and urethra. These pellets could cause many of the symptoms previously described with radiation irritation (proctitis). Rectal irritation can occur, though it is less frequent than with external-beam therapy.

Will I need a catheter in my bladder afterward?
Some physicians leave a catheter in overnight, though most patients are sent home the same day without requiring a catheter. Occasionally patients with urinary problems may have a catheter in for slightly longer.

If the cancer comes back after external-beam therapy, can I have radioactive seeds?

Not usually. When the maximum amount of radiation has been delivered to the rectal wall just behind the prostate, no additional radiation is permitted. To insert radioactive pellets into the prostate at that stage of treatment might increase the dose to the rectal wall beyond the amount that can be safely tolerated. In certain situations, however, some men can have seeds placed even after external beam. I have had this done for a few patients with good results.

Can these seeds be used for very large prostates?
In general, radioactive seeds are best for small to moderate-size prostates. If you have a very large prostate, you should talk to your radiation doctor and consider other treatment options.

What if my doctor is concerned that the cancer may have grown outside the prostate gland itself?
Then you are not a candidate for radioactive seeds. They are intended for those cancers confined (localized) within the prostate gland.

Can I have the seed treatment if I have had a TURP before?
Yes, but it is harder to do. The TURP is intended to reduce the blockage from an enlarged prostate by scooping out much of the tissue, leaving just a shell of tissue behind. The removal of tissue distorts and changes the normal prostate anatomy, making it more difficult to insert seeds accurately in the remaining tissue.

Will I be radioactive after seed therapy?
No, there will be a tiny amount of radiation given off by the seeds but not enough to be a threat to anyone, with the precautions as previously noted about pregnant women and small children and babies.

Will my urine or semen be radioactive?
No, neither will be.

What if I don't like the side effects of the seeds later on?
Usually the side effects will gradually subside over time. There are some medications that can help control side effects if they occur. Remember, the seeds can't be removed.

When can I go back to work?
You can usually safely return to work within a few days.

When can I resume activities like golf, tennis and exercising?
You can safely resume most activities within a few days. By then, you should be feeling better.

When can I resume sexual activity after the seeds are placed?
You should abstain for about four to six weeks. Then use a condom for the first few months.

Who does radioactive seed implantation?
This is done most often by radiation therapists, but a urologist may also be involved. In some locations, the urologist may actually do the procedure and simply use the radiation therapist to help with the radiation dose calculations and preparation. Quite often there is a team of doctors who routinely work together. The key point is that the more experienced the doctor, the better the results and the fewer complications you will have.

How soon will I know if the seed treatment worked?
You will have to wait several months at least, if not up to a year or more, watching the PSA test results. As long as the PSA continues to go down gradually, we feel good that cancer cells are being killed. The radiation doesn't kill all cancer cells immediately.

Are there any new techniques?

Researchers are experimenting with three-dimensional MRI real-time inter-stitial therapy to be even more precise with seed placement. Preliminary re-sults are very promising.

What about temporary seeds?

Called "high dose rate brachytherapy," small tubes are placed into the prostate, and radioactive seeds are placed into these tubes for a predetermined period of time and then the seeds and tubes are removed. About 15% of brachytherapy uses this technique.

RADICAL PROSTATECTOMY— A SURGICAL SOLUTION

21

For selected patients, most prostate-cancer specialists believe that *radical prostatectomy* offers a better chance for long-term survival and a longer time without return of the cancer than do the more conservative treatment options, such as radiation, hormone treatment or active surveillance.

Radical prostatectomy is a surgical operation in which the entire prostate gland and adjacent glands are removed surgically for the treatment of prostate cancer. It is one of the most common operations being performed today by urologists.

Why have I read that the surgery is not needed for prostate cancer?
A small but vocal group of physicians is asking that we stop doing the surgeries until we have definite proof that surgery will guarantee a survival advantage for each and every patient.

We know that prostate cancer is a disease whose response to treatment, whether or not it works, is measured in ten to fifteen years or more. That being true, do we doom many tens of thousands of men to an early death while we wait for new facts that may be a decade or more away? Most studies have shown that early detection and treatment have resulted in definite survival advantages for men who want to live without cancer. Surgery can be

> **?**
>
> *Is surgery a good option for every man with prostate cancer?*
>
> Surgery is definitely not for everyone. Surgery is not for men who will not live long enough to see the benefits. This is why we tend to look at surgery as an *option* for younger men. As a man grows older, his risks associated with surgery go up, his recovery is slower, the rate of potential complications increases and, in general, the risks begin to outweigh the benefits. Remember that age is based on the year you were born and also your general health.

very effective and should be reserved for those men who we believe can be helped by removing the cancer from the body.

Does early detection make a difference for prostate cancer?

For almost all other cancers, early detection and removal is associated with better survival. This is also true for prostate cancer. Studies suggest that the death rate from prostate cancer may be dropping for the first time, as a result of early detection and curative treatments like radical prostatectomy.

Is this a major or minor operation?

A radical prostatectomy is considered a *major* operation. It requires a significant hospitalization and has some potentially serious risks.

What is the goal of the surgery?

The intent of a radical prostatectomy is to remove the cancer from your body before it has had a chance to spread and potentially reduce your quality of life and life span. Some specialists perform a radical prostatectomy when cancer has already spread outside the gland, with the hope of reducing the amount of cancer cells remaining in your body. They believe it is then easier for your body's immune system, assisted by medications and treatments, to work more effectively. However, there are real and unavoidable risks with the surgery. It is a question of balancing the possible benefits with the potential risks.

Who is a candidate for this operation?

I use three requirements to determine who is a candidate for radical prostatectomy and who should consider this as a reasonable option.

1. The patient must have prostate cancer that is hoped to be *confined* to
    the prostate. Though there are a few experts who think otherwise, most
    agree the goal of the operation is to remove *all* the cancer from your
    body.

2. The patient should be able to safely undergo an operation requiring
    general anesthesia.

3. The patient should have a life expectancy long enough to see the
    benefits of surgery, usually seven to ten years or more.

*Because I meet the candidate guidelines, does that mean I should have
this operation?*

No. It only means this is a *reasonable option* for you to consider. I believe
that if you have a long life expectancy ahead of you and it seems the cancer
is potentially curable, then the surgery may be your best treatment choice.
But surgery may not be right for everyone. Lifestyle, risks and family com-
mitments may all impact on what choice is best for you.

How soon should I have surgery?

You should wait at least six to eight weeks after your biopsies to allow all of
the swelling and inflammation around the prostate to resolve. This will make
the surgery much easier and safer. Don't delay indefinitely either.

*What if the biopsies or PSA levels suggest that I have a high-grade or
large cancer? Can I still have my prostate gland removed?*

Yes. In certain instances, especially with young men, radical surgery can be
used even if we know it alone may not be curative. This type of "step" combination approach allows for the best of each treatment, especially for high-
risk cancers. Sometimes we go ahead with surgery, knowing there is a chance
it may be curative, but if not, then we can always add on hormone or radiation therapy afterward. I have seen amazing survival results in selected men
with aggressive cancer that had already spread to the nearby lymph nodes,

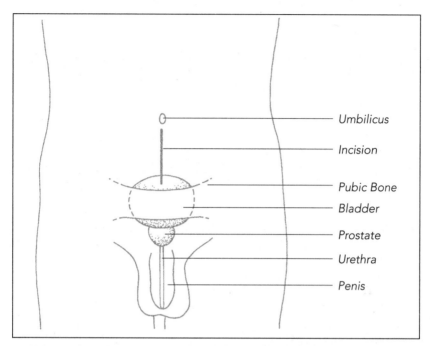

ABDOMINAL INCISION FOR RADICAL PROSTATECTOMY. In a radical retropubic prostatectomy, the prostate is removed through a lower abdominal incision that extends from the top of the pubic bone, just above the penis, up to the umbilicus (belly button).

after undergoing radical surgery with hormone therapy to follow. The thought is that the surgery removed almost all the cancer, making other treatments more effective.

Should I use a predicting table to tell if surgery is right for me?

No. You can use them (see page 112) to help add information for your discussions with your urologist. I often find that the tables simply tell me what I know from my experience and common sense. Some experts like to refer to tables to predict the likelihood for success or failure of surgery, based on the PSA, grade of the cancer or volume of cancer in the biopsies. Predictive tables are nice for publications, great for predicting results with large groups of people, but difficult to use and flawed with individual patients. These tables are helpful tools, but should not be used to make specific treatment recommendations for an individual. Dr. Partin at Johns

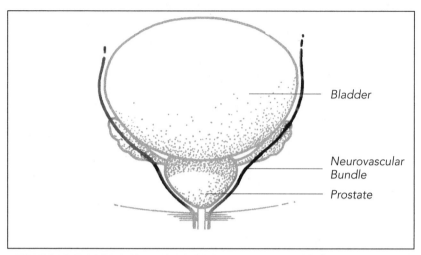

NERVES ALONGSIDE THE PROSTATE. Nerves responsible for erections travel alongside the prostate and can easily be damaged or cut during prostate removal. Nerve damage can also occur during radiation.

Hopkins himself told me he never intended for these tables to dictate an individual's care. They are to be used to discuss options and scenarios.

Surgical Options: Open vs. Laparoscopic, Retropubic vs. Perineal Approach

The most commonly used technique for radical prostatectomy in the United States is called the *retropubic approach*. An incision is made from just below the belly button to the top of the pubic bone. (See diagram on page 169.) The surgeon then exposes and removes the lymph nodes that drain the prostate. The prostate gland is then removed. The other open surgical option is a *perineal prostatectomy*. A perineal approach allows for removal of the prostate through an incision under the scrotum. (See diagram on page 171.)

Are the lymph nodes that drain the prostate analyzed?
It is common at the time of the radical prostatectomy for your doctor to remove and evaluate the lymph nodes. These nodes are then analyzed by a pathologist, often during the surgery, to see if any cancer has spread from the prostate. This is done to be certain that the appropriate treatment has been chosen.

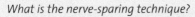

What is the nerve-sparing technique?

The nerve-sparing technique for prostate removal is based on a better understanding of the location of nerves that are responsible for penile erections. When these nerves are not removed or damaged during surgery, some men are later able to regain erections. It can take up to 12 to 18 months or more for erections to return.

Does everyone need to have the lymph nodes removed?

No, if the cancer is felt to be small-volume, low-grade and confined to the prostate, many surgeons do not perform a lymph-node dissection.

Do you risk leaving cancer behind if you leave the nerves intact?

It is generally accepted to leave only the nerves on the side opposite the cancer to be certain that all the cancer *is* removed. (See diagram on page 172.) Much depends on the cancer itself and the anatomy once we are in surgery, as well as the skill, experience and track record of the surgeon.

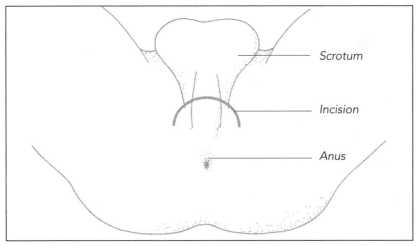

PERINEAL INCISION FOR RADICAL PROSTATECTOMY. In a radical perineal prostatectomy, the prostate is removed through an incision under the scrotum, with the legs elevated.

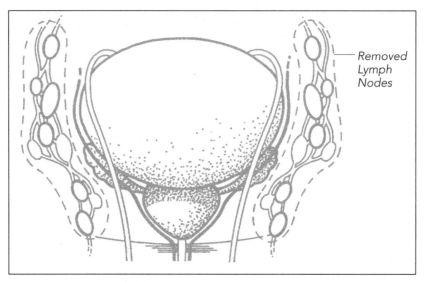

LYMPH-NODE DISSECTION. Lymph nodes that drain from the prostate are removed and analyzed by the pathologist to see if cancer has spread.

What is the advantage of the retropubic approach?

The main advantage of the retropubic approach is its easy access to the lymph nodes, nerves and blood vessels that are adjacent to the prostate. The lymph nodes can be removed at the same time and through the same incision used for the prostate-gland removal. Also, nerves can be identified and preserved and blood vessels controlled.

What is the benefit of the perineal approach?

The *perineal approach* to remove the prostate is made using an incision under the scrotum, in front of the rectum. The prostate is then separated from surrounding tissues and removed. (See diagram on page 171.) The perineal prostatectomy has always had the reputation of being less traumatic to the body, with a quicker recovery and less pain. With advances in the retropubic approach, these past advantages of the perineal technique are less an issue but are still being debated.

The advantages of one technique over the other are less clear today. The perineal approach is excellent for obese men where using the retropubic approach would be next to impossible because of the large lower abdominal

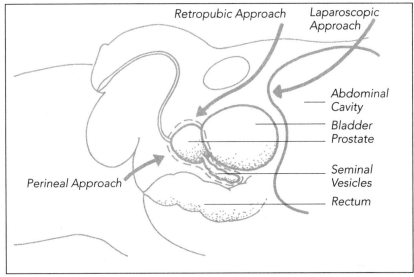

Retropubic Approach

Laparoscopic Approach

Abdominal Cavity

Bladder

Prostate

Seminal Vesicles

Rectum

Perineal Approach

COMPARISON OF SURGICAL APPROACHES FOR PROSTATECTOMY. Retropubic approach for radical prostatectomy is behind the pubic bone and in front of the bladder. Perineal radical prostatectomy allows for access to the prostate through the perineum. Laparoscopic approach is through the abdominal cavity to access the prostate.

wall. The key is to choose a surgeon who is skilled and experienced at whatever technique he or she prefers. The specific technique used is not as important as the skill of your surgeon.

What is a laparoscopic (lap) prostate removal?

This is an exciting and evolving technique to remove the prostate with only "Band-Aid" incisions. The prostate is removed through multiple fiber-optic probes placed into the abdomen. This is a very technically difficult and challenging technique.

How is this different from a robotic laparoscopic surgery?

Robotic laparoscopic surgery uses a 3-D da Vinci robot to allow for better and more precise movements during a lap prostatectomy; this procedure is commonly known as a *da Vinci laparoscopic robotic prostatectomy.* The surgeon actually sits at a large computer console next to the patient, and is able to see and move the laparoscopic instruments through the use of the robot. The

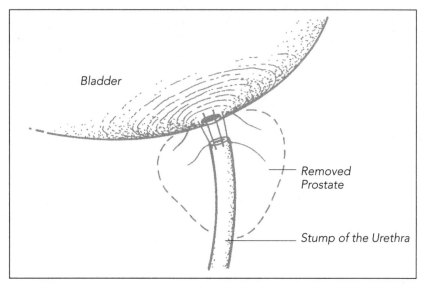

ATTACHMENT OF URETHRA TO BLADDER. After removal of the prostate
gland, the stump of the urethra is sewn back to the opening in the bladder neck.

use of the robot allows for natural motions in otherwise difficult-to-reach
areas within the pelvis and makes precise placement of stitches possible. Recovery can be a bit faster after robotic prostatectomy.

World-class expert Dr. Sanjay Ramakumar from Tucson, Arizona, describes the procedure as technically demanding but worth the effort. He explains that a well-performed laparoscopic robotic prostatectomy can offer
excellent results with reduced blood loss because of the improved magnifica-
tion. Currently this technique is performed by trained specialists at many
hospitals and referral centers.

*I have heard that the lap robotic prostatectomy has a steep learning
curve. What does this mean?*
With any new technique, it takes time or experiences to master the new chal-
lenges and skills required. This is what is referred to as "the learning curve."
The longer the learning curve, the longer it takes to master those necessary
skills. With a lap prostatectomy, it takes an average of 50 surgeries for a surgeon to perfect his skills. Using these new technologies will not make your
doctor a better surgeon. To do a lap robotic prostatectomy correctly, the doc-

tor must be a good surgeon and understand the techniques of prostate removal. Robotics will allow a good surgeon to be able to perform laparoscopic prostatectomies more efficiently and with consistent outcomes.

Is one approach better than another?

No. It is most important for the surgeon to do whichever technique he or she feels is best for you, the one he or she can perform best and with the least complications. Each surgeon tends to have a favorite technique, one he or she was probably trained to do and perform most often. In competent hands, it really doesn't make a difference which approach is used. The main factor should be what treatment is best for you. Once you decide on surgical removal, then you should allow the urologist you trust to advise you on the best technique for you.

How does robotic prostatectomy compare with open prostatectomy as far as impotence or incontinence?

The rates of impotence and urine control are the same. The most important factor in minimizing complications is the skill and expertise of your surgeon, whatever technique is performed.

Why don't all urologists do a robotic prostatectomy?

Each doctor has his or her own skills and experience. Some surgeons are very competent with excellent cancer removal rates, nerve preservation and very low complications with an open prostatectomy. Again, it is not the specific technique your doctor chooses that is important—it is that he or she is skilled, is experienced and has a good track record.

How long does a robotic prostatectomy take?

About two to three hours on average, slightly longer than an open prostatectomy.

How many robotic prostatectomies should my doctor do to be good?

As with any surgery, whether open or laparoscopic, you will see better results, have better cure and encounter fewer complications with more experience. In general, whatever the technique, your doctor should perform one or two cases a week on average. That being said, numbers alone are not enough. Some highly skilled surgeons can do far fewer prostatectomies and offer great results while other less talented doctors can do many more and still have poor results.

What if my doctor has not performed many robotic prostatectomies?

This technique requires extra training and experience for the doctor to be able to offer the same level of care as an open prostatectomy. In general, your doctor should have performed at least 50 lap robotic prostatectomies for his or her results to be as good as those of a skilled open procedure. Likewise, the hospital and operating room team should be regularly performing these procedures to obtain and maintain the skills needed to assist your urologist.

What can go wrong with a laparoscopic prostatectomy?

This operation is very challenging and not easily mastered by everyone. Your surgeon operates through small incisions, using a video camera and special extended instruments. The three-dimensional benefits of open surgery are lost.

During this procedure, there is always a chance that one of the large nerves that passes through the pelvis can be cut or damaged. These nerves are important for certain movements of the legs.

Likewise, blood vessels can be torn. If nerve or blood-vessel damage occurs, the surgeon will have to stop the laparoscopic surgery and make an abdominal incision to control the bleeding or repair the cut nerve.

How is the urethra attached to the bladder after the prostate is removed?

A radical prostatectomy leaves a small hole at the bottom of the bladder where the prostate used to be located. The cut and unattached urethra also remains. Stitches are then placed through the urethral stump to the bladder neck, a catheter is placed into the bladder and the bladder neck and urethra are brought together. The catheter is usually left in seven to ten days on average. (See diagram on page 174.) Infrequently a man will describe slight penile shortening.

Is a prostatectomy an easy operation to perform?
No. It probably is one of the more challenging operations to learn correctly. Even when a surgeon has the skills mastered, it still can be a challenge.

What can make the operation more difficult?
Men who are quite obese and have a very wide abdominal wall or perineum force us to work in a deeper hole through a narrower opening. Some men have particularly deep and narrow pelvic bones, which can make the procedure more challenging. Occasionally, the prostate can have very large blood vessels adjacent to the top of the gland. And as if these aren't enough obstacles, very large prostates or prostates in men who have had previous surgery (such as a TURP) can be difficult to remove. Laparoscopic robotic prostatectomy is probably better for obese men, because the extra fat can actually be an advantage in skilled hands.

If another surgeon is faster, does that mean he is better?
No. Quality of the results, patient satisfaction and keeping problems and complications to a minimum are the only factors that should determine how good a surgeon is.

The history of the fast surgeon dates back to a time when there was no anesthesia. The faster the surgeon could amputate a limb, the less pain you had. Fortunately, we now have anesthesia. We can take our time and do operations carefully and accurately.

Will I still be fertile after my prostate is removed?
You will not be able to father children the normal way. The surgery removes many of the essential glands and tubes that bring together all the necessary ingredients for the sperm to live and survive. Though your body still makes sperm, there is no way they can get out naturally. There are several techniques where we can extract sperm to be used.

Preparation for Surgery

What things do I have to do in preparation for surgery?

There are a number of routine preoperative tests and treatments we do to reduce the risks of surgery, to get you as ready as you can be. The reason for the following procedures is to minimize risks that cannot be eliminated from surgery.

One risk is bleeding during surgery. To help lower the risk of bleeding, we request that you stop taking aspirin and aspirin-containing products for ten days before your scheduled surgery. Some of the most common over-the-counter brand-name products containing aspirin are AlkaSeltzer, Anacin, Bayer, Aspergum, Empirin, Bufferin, Ecotrin and Ascriptin. If you take ibuprofen, Advil, Motrin, Anaprox or similar anti-inflammatory medications, these also should be stopped for at least three to five days before your surgery date. If you are not sure about any of your medications, ask your doctor. If you were put on aspirin by your doctor because of heart or blood problems, then you need to get permission from that doctor to stop the aspirin. Please stop vitamin E, fish oil supplements or garlic tablets several weeks before surgery.

Another risk, though rare, is tearing of the rectal wall adjacent to the prostate. In the old days the torn area would be sewn up and a colostomy would be made to divert the feces away from the healing area of the rectal wall. Three months later the colostomy would be closed, and your normal bowel function would return.

ANTI-INFLAMMATORY MEDICATIONS

Advil	Feldene	Mefenamic Acid
Aleve	Flurbiprofen	Motrin
Anaprox	Ibuprofen	Naprosyn
Ansaid	Indocin	Naproxen
Clinoril	Ketorolac	Nuprin
Daypro	Lodine	Nalfon
Diclofenac	Meclofenamate	Oxaprozin
Etodolac	Meclomen	

CLEAR-LIQUID DIET

Apple Juice	Gatorade
Grape Juice	Tea
Cranberry Juice	Coffee
Carbonated Soda	Clear broth

The fear with this injury is the development of an abscess or pocket of infection. To eliminate or dramatically reduce the odds for an abscess, some doctors put you through a *bowel-prep*. With a bowel-prep, your intestines will be relatively cleaned out. You will also be given antibiotics to reduce the risks of infection. Because you can become dehydrated after this cleansing, be sure to drink lots of water, clear liquids or Gatorade afterward.

You will be admitted to the hospital the morning of surgery, so you will do this bowel preparation and take antibiotics at home the day before surgery. Because the complication of rectal-wall injury is so rare, many urologists don't believe it is necessary to have a bowel-prep.

To reduce your risks of blood clots, many doctors use *pneumatic sequential stockings*—special inflatable stockings that intermittently squeeze and release around your calves and legs, forcing blood to circulate to reduce the risk of clots. These stockings are worn even if you are not moving and are asleep during surgery. You will be directed to use these stockings for a few days after surgery.

Does pretreatment with hormone shots actually cause the cancer to shrink?

There is much debate on this question. Some experts have thought that with hormone pretreatment we could *downstage* the cancer, or convert it from a stage with cancer growing *outside* the gland to a lesser stage with the cancer confined *within* the prostate.

However, recent studies don't support this belief, so most experts don't do downstaging. We do know that hormone shots will cause the prostate itself to shrink in size but may increase the scarring around the prostate and actually make it harder to remove. This pretreatment doesn't seem to improve survival.

Anesthesia

Is there significant pain with surgery?
Surprisingly, no. Most men are pleased how good they feel afterward. Many tell me they never had any real pain, not even enough for a single over-the-counter pain pill.

These days, with the use of epidural anesthesia, new medications and PCA pumps, pain is not usually an issue. Not that long ago, if you had pain, you would have to ring for the nurses, who would then give you a shot of morphine or Demerol. Now, just before surgery, many men have an epidural catheter placed to control any pain or discomfort.

What is epidural anesthesia?
Epidural anesthesia is the same anesthesia that many women have during childbirth. This is a type of anesthesia in which a small amount of a potent narcotic drips directly into the fluid that surrounds the spinal cord. This results in blockage of all pain, but still allows normal sensation and muscle function. It is a rare patient who can't have an epidural placed. I almost insist on one with every case, because it makes the postoperative time so well tolerated.

There are some new methods where the epidural is used for only a day or two, and then a non-narcotic is given to control any pain. Some surgeons are using this powerful non-narcotic alone with excellent results.

What is a PCA pump?
PCA stands for *patient-controlled analgesia*. A PCA pump is a device attached to the intravenous-fluid line. Whenever you feel pain, you simply push a button and a small amount of narcotic is injected into your bloodstream. The machine has internal controls to prevent an overdose and limit the maximum dose.

How is an epidural different from a spinal anesthetic?
The spinal anesthetic blocks the ability to feel and use the legs. The epidural anesthetic can block just pain.

How does an epidural work?
An epidural works by putting the anesthetic medication around the nerves that transmit the sensation of pain up from the lower abdomen and legs.

What if I've had previous back surgery?
Scarring from a previous back surgery can be a problem if the doctor is unable to place the epidural catheter into the correct location because of it.

What are some of the side effects of an epidural anesthetic?
The most common side effect is itching, which can be treated. Rare risks include breathing difficulty or infection.

What if my surgeon doesn't want to use an epidural?
Some urologists are using a powerful non-narcotic medication with very good results. Many men describe minimal discomfort and are going home in just a few days.

Will I be asleep during the surgery if I have an epidural?
Yes, most patients are put under a general anesthesia so the patient is in deep sleep and totally unaware of proceedings during surgery, whatever method of pain control is used after surgery.

Will herbs or supplements interact with the anesthetic medications?
Possibly. In general, it is wise to stop *all* herbs and supplements two weeks before surgery, to prevent a surprise interaction with the anesthetic medications.

During the Surgery

Can I have my hernia fixed at the same time I have prostate surgery?
Yes. If you have a hernia that may need to be repaired, be sure to ask your doctor and talk to a general surgeon as well. It is important to tell your urologist so he or she can coordinate this with the general surgeon. Although the urologist can do the hernia repair, general surgeons do most of them.

Can you remove just the one side of the prostate that has cancer?

No. Even if the biopsies and/or ultrasound show that the cancer appears to be on just one side of the prostate, the pathologist will often find that the cancer really is in multiple locations on both sides. For this reason, it is not safe to consider a partial prostate removal.

In addition, technically it would be almost impossible to remove only one side completely. It is fairly easy to sew the cut end of the urethra onto the bottom end of the bladder after the prostate is removed. To leave one side of the prostate would make the operation very difficult and make the reconnection less water-tight and more likely to leak.

Does surgery on the prostate cause cancer cells to spread?

No, there is no evidence or research indicating that cancer spreads with surgery. When we do this operation, we do it in a way to keep the gland and surrounding tissues as intact as we can. Cancer cells are constantly leaving the gland and entering into the bloodstream, and this occurs during surgery as well. But no studies have ever shown that surgery results in increased cancer spread. Most of these cells are destroyed quickly by the body's immune system.

Do you examine the prostate gland when it is removed?

Yes, the entire specimen is analyzed and cut into tiny slices. Key pieces are reviewed under the microscope by a pathologist who will determine the type, grade and extent of cancer. Information regarding the volume of the cancer as well as the status of the lymph nodes will be reported. This information allows the urologist to decide if additional treatments are needed, and which would be best.

Prostate Evaluation During Surgery

What if you are concerned during surgery that the cancer has spread?

We can always send tiny pieces of tissue to the pathologists to see if cancer is present. We also send the lymph nodes, which can be analyzed immediately

Can my wife visit me in the recovery room after my prostatectomy?

Not usually. Most recovery rooms are not set up to allow visitors. They are often very large rooms with a number of nursing stations and beds placed between these stations. It would be awkward if you walked right in among men and women in different stages of recovering from surgery. Usually the nurses will let your family know how you are doing and when you are transferred to your regular room.

by *frozen-section analysis* if they are suspicious to be sure the cancer has not spread.

What is a frozen section?

This is how pathologists look quickly at tissue sent in during your surgery to see whether cancer is present. A frozen section is most commonly performed on the lymph nodes to be sure there is no evidence of cancer spread before proceeding to remove the prostate itself.

Rather than routine processing and analysis, which can take a day or more, frozen-section analysis allows the pathologist to freeze the tissue very quickly with liquid nitrogen. Tiny, thin slices of the frozen tissue are then cut off and examined for cancer.

Although a rapid procedure, the freezing process can distort what is seen and make it less accurate than the routine analysis, called *permanent section.*

Recovery Room

How long will I be in recovery?

It is common for a patient to be in recovery for an hour or two or even more after a radical prostatectomy.

Hospitalization

Will I need to stay in the intensive care unit?

Probably not. In my experience, it is a rare patient who needs more nursing care and observation than is offered on the regular urology floor. If there are medical concerns, your doctor may place you in the intensive care unit (ICU) for the first night. After a radical prostatectomy, patients usually go to the ICU not because they are very ill, but because they have the potential for problems.

The ICU provides close one-on-one nursing and monitoring. These rare patients may have significant heart or lung problems, or perhaps there were some irregular heartbeats during surgery that we want to observe more closely.

If you are so ill from a nonurologic problem as to require ICU care after surgery, then perhaps you really aren't a good candidate for surgery in the first place. This is something to consider and discuss with your doctor.

In the ICU, visitation by family members is fairly limited. Friends are usually not allowed. Traffic and noise must be kept to a minimum.

How long will I be in the hospital?

You will usually spend between two and three days in the hospital, including the day of surgery (one to two days for perineal prostatectomy). Most patients go home on the second postoperative day. After laparoscopic prostatectomy, you will probably go home the next day.

How soon you are discharged depends on how quickly you recuperate. When your bowels "wake up" after surgery and you begin eating a regular diet, then you usually are discharged. Unlike in the past, it is generally considered best to get out of the hospital as soon as you are able. You are better off walking and being active than lying in a hospital bed, waiting for nurses to come in and walk you.

Another reason to go home is to avoid infection. Despite the best handwashing in the world, hospitals are known for harboring dangerous and difficult-to-treat infections. The sooner you get out, the better you will be.

How long do I have to stay in bed while in the hospital?
We don't want you to stay in bed. We want you to get up and walk around. The more you are up and around, the quicker your recovery. In my practice, I ask you to walk about two times the night after surgery, and then at least four to six times every day afterward. The bed should really be the place where you go only to sleep or take a nap.

Is it better to take one long walk or several small walks?
The goal is to get you up and moving. With this in mind, more frequent short walks are much better than a long walk.

Do I have to wait for a nurse to help me?
The first few times you walk, you will need to have a nurse or assistant accompany you. You probably will have several lines and tubes attached to your body. The nurses will get these positioned so you can walk. Sometimes you can get a little dizzy, nauseated or light-headed at first, so it's always better to have someone with you who can support you and help you back to bed.

What can I do to reduce dizziness?
When you get up to walk, do it slowly and sit on the edge of the chair or bed for a few minutes before you stand up.

Should I bring my own medications to the hospital?
Yes. It is very important that we are able to continue your regular medications. Bring them in the original containers to help the hospital pharmacist identify each medication.

Will my primary-care doctor be at surgery?
Not usually. Some family practitioners like to assist with surgery on their own patients, but this is infrequent.

Will my primary-care doctor need to see me after surgery?
If you need to be seen for other serious medical problems or concerns, yes. Usually, however, it isn't necessary. You should at least call after you get home to let your primary-care doctor know you are home and doing well. If you

don't need to be seen, then a follow-up visit with him or her can be on your routine schedule. If you do have any problems at all after surgery, you should contact your urologist and primary-care doctor right away.

Controversy: Quality of Life vs. Longevity

There is much debate on the quality of life associated with each of the treatments for prostate cancer. We want to know if the patient is happy with his choice of treatment and the potential complications, such as urinary incontinence or impotence.

I have found that most men are indeed pleased with the treatment they have chosen. My personal philosophy and emphasis has always been to provide the necessary information so my patients can select the option they feel is best. I want them to consider the potential risks and complications from their choice.

If you are told by someone else what you are going to do, then I suspect you will be less tolerant of anything less than perfect results. On the other hand, if you make your own decision with complete awareness of the risks, then in my experience you are far more likely to accept whatever happens as a result of your choice.

Isn't it easy to assess quality of life?
All individuals interpret quality of life differently. My patients' perceptions of their problems after surgery have always amazed me.

I recall one man who had a very aggressive, advanced cancer that required radiation after surgery. Subsequently, he became incontinent of urine, yet he remained positive and optimistic about the future. He was very happy and appreciative of my services.

This man's attitude contrasts with a patient who, after much deliberation, finally decided to have a prostatectomy. He was clearly unhappy with what he felt was his only real option, but he went ahead with surgery. Six months later, he came in for a follow-up appointment, very disturbed and depressed over his continued incontinence. On further questioning, it turned out that about once every few weeks, if he lifted a heavy object when his bladder was full, he might leak a few drops of urine. He was upset about his horrible situation.

He was unhappy because he believed he had no choice about treating his cancer, even though his results weren't nearly as bad as he perceived. At the same time, the first man was thrilled that his cancer was under control and that he was able to live and enjoy the day-to-day joys of life, despite the nuisance of leakage.

My point is, quality of life is not something you can standardize for all people. Each patient has to decide if he is happy with how things turned out. I suspect a fair number of men are unhappy, not so much with any problem but more with the fact that they had cancer and required a treatment they really didn't want to have.

I try to tell my patients they need to look at the cards they are dealt and make a decision based on those cards. At least they have choices, although not what they might prefer. I remind them there are men who don't have the options they have.

Controversy: Long-Term Benefits vs. Potential Risks

Most urology experts believe that for selected men, radical prostatectomy offers the potential for better long-term survival, based on this important

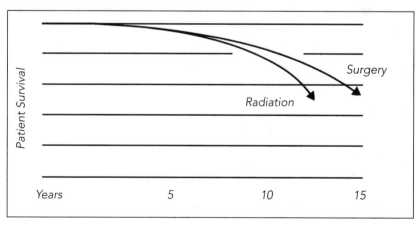

SURVIVAL AFTER SURGERY VERSUS AFTER RADIATION. Patients who have had surgery have survival advantages after seven to ten years.

observation: The success rate of radical prostatectomy and radiation is roughly the same for the first seven to ten years. After seven to ten years, the success rate of prostatectomy is higher compared with radiation.

I tell my patients, "If you don't think you're going to be around in seven to ten years, then don't take the risks of surgery. You can choose a more conservative choice, such as radiation, that can provide essentially the same results with significantly fewer risks."

There are those who believe that prostatectomy has not been clearly proven to offer advantages over radiation therapy or no treatment at all. Many long-term studies are under way to compare these options. Until we have conclusive data, I believe that it is important to base our decisions on current clinical experience.

The psychological benefits of surgery are also important, although difficult to describe. For some men, it is important to know that the cancer is out of their bodies and in a jar in the pathologist's back office.

Other men are willing to undergo less aggressive therapy in order to avoid the potential risks of surgery. Your personal feelings about the risks and benefits of surgery as compared with radiation therapy are very important and should be considered when discussing your options. You must choose the treatment you are most comfortable with.

RISKS AND COMPLICATIONS OF RADICAL PROSTATECTOMY

22

E very treatment for prostate cancer carries the potential of certain undesirable side effects or complications, which sometimes cannot be
avoided, even in the best of hands. Each person is different, each cancer is different and every patient responds differently to each treatment. You
should realize that there are potential problems. Most men, however, will
experience none of these complications.

The most common potential problems are *impotence*, or the lack of penile
erections, and *urinary incontinence*, or the leaking of urine. These special
problems are discussed in detail in later chapters.

Other risks include *bleeding* during and after surgery, the development
of a *bladder-neck contracture, deep venous thrombosis, pulmonary emboli* and
urinary-tract infection.

Bleeding

Is there bleeding during surgery?
The prostate and adjacent structures are rich with multiple and often large
blood vessels. In the process of removing the prostate, it is possible to lose a

lot of blood. Bleeding is more likely if the prostate is very large, you have had prior hormone therapy or you have a general anesthesia.

How can there be bleeding after surgery?

If a clot breaks off a small artery or vein, bleeding can begin. This is quite rare. It's something urologists are aware of as a risk but rarely see. If the bleeding were significant, then you might need transfusions or possibly even a return to surgery to identify and stop whatever is bleeding.

Can I donate my own blood before surgery to reduce the need for a transfusion if bleeding does occur?

Maybe. Your doctor may ask you to donate blood in advance of surgery. Though unlikely, if you should need a transfusion, then your doctor can use your own blood. You can give one or two pints of blood each session, depending on the specific technique.

Your own blood is called *autologous blood.* Because it is uncommon to need your blood, many surgeons don't routinely require autologous donations. They feel that it lowers the threshold to need a transfusion. Their concern is that when you donate blood you might drop your starting blood count so you are more likely to need a transfusion. Others feel that the donation of blood ahead of time actually stimulates your own body's blood-production mechanism to move into full speed, which helps with your immediate recovery.

Can I donate my own blood ahead of time?

Yes, I offer my patients the option of donating one or two units of their blood. Called *autologous donations,* this blood is held only for its donor and can be given if a transfusion is required.

How often is a transfusion required?

This is variable, depending again on the surgeon and the volume of blood loss. Some surgeons may need to give blood on a regular basis if the blood loss is high. The average is about 5% of men nationally who need transfusions during and after surgery.

Can you recycle blood lost during surgery?
Yes, some urologists use a machine called a *cell saver* that takes the blood lost during the removal of the prostate and prepares and recycles the blood back to the patient.

Some doctors give a medicine that can actually stimulate the body to make more red blood cells. This is quite expensive.

How often do you have to give autologous blood to a patient?
It is the rare patient who needs some of his own blood back. I prefer to look at the autologous blood as an insurance policy so that if there is an unexpected problem, we'll have some of your own blood available.

Should I sign the hospital consent to allow for transfusion even if I've already given autologous blood?
Yes, definitely, you should give your doctor permission to administer blood products as needed. This must be signed in order for you to receive your own donated blood. In case of that rare situation when there is dramatic blood loss, you will have given your doctor permission to give you transfusions if it is felt necessary to save your life.

Every doctor is aware of the "unlikelihood" of the patient getting hepatitis or AIDS from a regular blood transfusion. This risk is very small and should be balanced with a sudden need for blood in an emergency situation.

If you have any questions, talk to your urologist before surgery. Express your concerns. For your own safety, don't sign "no" unless your urologist knows of your intentions ahead of time.

What do they do with the autologous blood that is not used?
The blood must be thrown away. It is drawn specifically for you. If not used, it must be discarded according to Red Cross guidelines.

Why can't I just get my blood back anyway?
There is always a tiny chance of a paperwork mistake, so it is considered acceptable to have an autologous donation only if you truly need the blood.

Can people donate blood for me?

Yes, they can. This is called *directed donation*. However, most often the blood types do not match closely enough to be used. Even if they do match, there is actually a higher risk for hepatitis and AIDS than from the general population of people who regularly donate blood. This is explained by the fact that there may be tremendous social and family pressure for a relative to donate blood even if he or she has had experiences in the past that may have increased the risk of picking up one of these diseases.

Bladder-Neck Contracture

What is a bladder-neck contracture?

This is scar tissue that forms at the bladder neck after surgery, where the urethra was sewn to the bladder. This can result in urination problems.

How do I know if I have developed a contracture?

Most men describe a weakened urinary stream with more and more difficulty urinating. Because the prostate is totally removed, you shouldn't have any significant problems with blockage. Any symptoms that suggest there may be a blockage should be evaluated further to be sure there is no scar tissue.

How common is bladder-neck contracture?

It is uncommon, but can occur in about one out of every twenty to thirty prostatectomies.

How are these evaluated and treated?

I identify bladder-neck contractures in my patients with an office cystoscopy. If I find a scar, I try to stretch it open in the office with metal dilators. Though uncomfortable for a few moments, it saves most men a trip to surgery under anesthesia. There may be bleeding after the scar is opened. Some men complain of increased urinary incontinence after the stretching procedure. This can be significant but is rarely permanent.

If simple stretching hasn't worked and surgery is required for a severe or recurrent scar tissue, I often just cut the scar open in two locations with a laser and leave a catheter in for about 24 hours. This is usually done successfully as an outpatient procedure under anesthesia. The main concern is the return of urinary incontinence after the scar is opened up.

Can the scar tissue come back?
Yes, occasionally some men will have a return of the scar, although this is uncommon. It can come back within a few weeks or perhaps years later.

Deep Venous Thrombosis (DVT) and Pulmonary Embolus (PE)

What is a DVT?
A *deep venous thrombosis* (*DVT*) is a blood clot that can develop in the veins of the legs or pelvis. Such clots can cause swelling of the leg. They are of concern because of the potential for breaking loose and floating up to the heart and lungs. If a clot breaks loose and reaches the heart and lungs, it is called a *pulmonary embolus* (*PE*).

How is a pulmonary embolus dangerous?
The pulmonary embolus may pass through the right side of the heart and be pumped at high pressure into the lungs. If large, it can totally block blood flow and result in an almost-instant drop of blood pressure. This would cause death almost instantaneously. This is one of the most common causes of sudden death after surgery. Fortunately, they are quite rare. Pulmonary emboli can occur days to weeks after surgery.

How can I avoid the risk of a pulmonary embolus or venous thrombosis?
To help reduce this potential risk, during surgery I use special stockings that inflate and deflate to keep the blood flowing through the veins. I get the patient up and walking the evening after surgery and frequently thereafter. I also have him use support stockings after surgery. Some specialists give blood

> ### RADICAL PROSTATECTOMY RISKS
>
> Impotence   Bladder-neck contracture
> Incontinence   Blood clots/heart attack
> Bleeding/transfusions   Need for additional treatments
> Infections

thinners or start aspirin after surgery to prevent these clots from forming. The key is movement. Lying in bed without moving is dangerous.

Not all blood clots break loose, and many cause only minor problems. It is the rare large clot that can be fatal. If you experience leg or calf swelling or pain after surgery, or if you have sudden chest pain or difficult/painful breathing, call your doctor *immediately*.

Other Complications

Are there any long-term complications to a lymph-node dissection?
Yes. Rarely, after surgical lymph-node removal, a lymphocele can develop.

What is a lymphocele?
A *lymphocele* is a pocket of lymphatic fluid that builds up in the pelvis, usually following the lymph-node dissection. This fluid can put pressure on surrounding tissues and organs and cause lower abdominal pressure or pain. If it becomes infected, you can become quite ill with fever, chills and severe abdominal pain.

Why does this pocket develop?
It develops because the normal drainage of lymph fluid is interrupted when the lymph nodes are removed.

How common is this complication?
This is fairly rare, occurring in only one or two men out of every one hundred operations performed. The incidence may actually be higher, but if the lymphocele is small and not causing any problem or symptoms, we wouldn't know about it.

How is a lymphocele treated?

If the lymphocele isn't large or isn't causing problems, I usually leave it alone. If it is causing pain or fever, then I drain the fluid. This is usually performed by a radiologist, often with the help of a CT scan or ultrasound.

Catheters or drains can be left in temporarily to continue the drainage. Rarely, surgery is required to open the pocket of fluid. Some urologists drain the fluid through laparoscopy with good results.

Can the lymphocele come back?

It can come back at any time in the future. Most are found within a few months to a year or more after surgery.

Can a nerve or blood vessel be cut or damaged during a lymph-node dissection?

This is rare, but sometimes there can be extensive scarring that can make it difficult to identify the adjacent nerve, which controls leg movement, or blood vessels. This nerve is different from the nerves that control erections.

What are the risks of getting pneumonia?

This complication is very uncommon, especially now that we get you up and walking right away after surgery. To reduce risks for lung infections, we also have you work on deep breathing during your hospital stay. I do not recall any of my patients developing pneumonia following radical prostatectomy.

Will I have an allergic reaction?

There is always a rare but possible chance you could have some kind of reaction to any medication you are given. If you are allergic to a medication, then we try not to give it unless the problem is felt to be life threatening and you need the antibiotic as a life saving measure.

Most allergic reactions are rashes, itching, hives or blisters. You could get a fever. More serious reactions include swelling of the lips and tongue or difficulty breathing. The most dangerous reaction is *anaphylaxis*, which can include sudden heart stoppage or halted breathing without warning. Fortunately, these serious reactions are extremely rare.

What are the risks of getting an infection?

Infection is always a possibility. To minimize this risk, we have you shower the night before with an antiseptic soap such as Hibiclens or Betadine. In addition, you will probably receive antibiotics at the time of surgery and for some time afterward.

The odds of developing a skin infection in the incision is very low. If you develop redness and tenderness or drainage of fluid, you should see your doctor and point out these changes.

Urinary-tract infections are always possible but unlikely. In my practice, I give antibiotics just at and after the time of surgery, then again around the time the catheter comes out. It is very rare to have a patient who develops an infection with this regimen. Some doctors will keep you on antibiotics as long as the catheter is in.

Can I get stomach ulcers after the surgery?

Over the years I can recall only one patient who developed stomach ulcers from the stress of surgery and the hospitalization.

If you have a history of stomach ulcers, it is important to tell your surgeon so he can consider giving you preventive medications.

What is the risk of a rectal injury requiring a colostomy?

As discussed in Chapter 21, this is a very rare complication that can occur when the back wall of the prostate is stuck to the front wall of the rectum. This can occur with extensive scarring or inflammation.

What about blood in the urine?

It is very normal to see some blood or even a few clots in the urine, on and off, while the catheter is in. The very delicate lining of the urethra can be irritated by the catheter and bleed. On occasion, some blood may even leak around the catheter.

Will the catheter prevent leaking of urine?

Most of the time, yes. There may be bladder spasms, where the bladder is irritated by the surgery and catheter, and tries to squeeze down. This squeezing can cause some urine to leak out. If this is painful or frequent, you should call your doctor.

Consent Form

Every surgery patient is asked to sign a *consent form*. See the Appendix for a copy of the radical prostatectomy consent form that I use. Every doctor's consent form is different, but this is one that points out many of the most serious problems that can occur during surgery. Always read a consent form carefully and make sure you understand it before you sign it. The consent is not intended to list every potential complication. Rather, it is a review of the most common and/or serious complications during or after surgery. Use the consent form to help you be a better and more informed patient. The more you know about what might go wrong, the better you will be at helping to identify potential problems early on.

RECOVERING AT HOME AFTER SURGERY

23

O nce the surgery is over, the responsibility for your recovery shifts from the doctor to you. The main goal after surgery is to get you back to your normal lifestyle as quickly as we can. There are some limitations during your initial recovery, but they shouldn't slow your ability to resume normal activities and regain your strength. How quickly you recover is a direct reflection of your motivation to bounce back.

It is important not to let surgery or recovery get in the way of your life. You may be slowed temporarily, but you shouldn't be stopped. As good as you feel after surgery, your body still is recovering from the stresses of an operation. You must be aware of this and allow yourself the flexibility to tolerate the limitations and changes you feel.

What can I expect regarding my short-term recovery?
Right after you arrive at home you will notice a lack of the energy level and endurance you had before surgery. When you have been up and around, you will find that you tire easily. At first, you might get up from a nap, shower and then need to lie down again. When the tiredness comes on, it hits you like a wall. You might feel weak, light-headed and possibly dizzy or even nauseated.

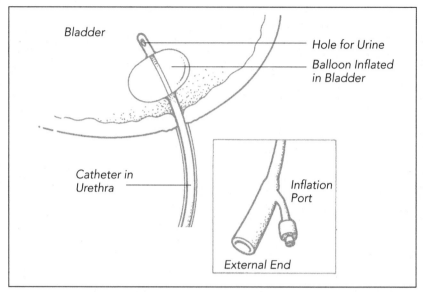

FOLEY CATHETER. This is a rubber or silicone catheter placed through the ure-thra into the bladder to allow constant urine drainage. The catheter is held in place by a balloon filled with water through an inflation port off to the side of the exter-nal end of the catheter. The external end drains into a collection bag.

How long is the recovery after a radical prostatectomy?
Most working men take off several weeks before returning to work. If you do heavy lifting or straining, it may take four to six weeks. We urge you to stay as active as possible. Strength doesn't return to the man who sits and watches TV, waiting to get better. You have to go out and earn it.

Catheter

Your doctor will send you home from the hospital with a *Foley catheter* in place. A Foley catheter is a hollow tube that is placed into the bladder during surgery to provide continuous urine drainage. It is held in place with an inflated balloon and connected to a drainage bag, which should be emptied regularly.

Will the catheter bother me?
As time goes by, the catheter will become an increasing nuisance. It is per-fectly normal to have occasional leakage of urine around the catheter, often

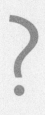

How long does the catheter need to stay in?

The average time for the catheter to remain is about one to two weeks, depending on the technique of surgery. This allows the area of the urethra sewn to the bladder neck to heal. If we took it out too soon, it would increase the risk of urinary incontinence. There's not much reason to leave it in longer.

without warning. You may have occasional bladder spasms, which usually go away over time.

What are bladder spasms?

Bladder spasms are a squeezing down of the bladder with a cramping, lower abdominal pain that usually goes away in a few minutes. It can come on suddenly or gradually build up. Your bladder does not tolerate the irritation of the catheter and balloon. Therefore, your bladder is trying to rid itself of the irritation by squeezing it out. I usually consider this a good sign of quick return of bladder function.

How can I stop the spasms?

Your doctor can help reduce the frequency and intensity of spasms by prescribing medications such as Detrol LA, Ditropan XL, Enablex or Urispas. If you are on such medication, ask your doctor when it is to be stopped. I usually stop the medication about 24 to 48 hours before the catheter is removed. The good news is that most often the spasms reduce and even go away within a few days.

What can I do to reduce problems with the catheter?

First, it's important to keep the area clean at the end of your penis where the catheter comes out. Wash the area with soap and water at least once or twice each day. You can also put a small dab of over-the-counter antibiotic ointment just at the opening. This not only will reduce the risk of developing an infection but also will reduce discomfort from the catheter sticking to the skin.

To keep the catheter from tugging on your penis, I recommend you attach the drainage bag with a safety pin to the elastic on your underwear.

Will I get an infection with the catheter in so long?
Probably not. You may get what is called *colonization,* where germs are present (they colonize) on the catheter and in the urine. But they have not progressed enough to cause an infection or symptoms. Just having germs on the catheter is not bad and does not require treatment. If you get a fever or the bladder spasms increase, call your doctor.

Exercise

What can I do to speed my recovery?
To overcome this reduced strength, you need to really push yourself. As I tell my patients, you can't just lie in bed and wait for your strength to return. You need to be up and active.

The more walking you do, the better and more quickly you'll recover. Frequent short walks are better than one long walk. If your house or apartment is too small for exercise, or if the weather outside is not good for a walk, then go to an indoor shopping mall. There you don't have to worry about the weather. You'll find plenty of places to sit if you get tired or need a drink or something to eat.

No other exercise is as good for your recovery as walking. Treadmills are also fine to use, but keep it fairly flat and slow and just try to put in the time.

How will I know if I've pushed myself too far?
During a walk, you may find yourself suddenly weak and tired, perhaps even nauseated and flushed. This is your body's way of letting you know you pushed yourself a little too far. You will notice that your strength and endurance are not what they were before surgery. But with work and patience, you'll be surprised how quickly you will recover. Often a midday nap or two is all you need for a while.

When can I walk after surgery?
You should be walking regularly even before you leave the hospital. When you go home, you should continue to walk about as much as you feel you

> *How often should I walk?*
>
> **?**
>
> It is probably smart to walk four to six times each day. Each time you walk, you should always walk a little farther than you feel comfortable doing. Keep pushing just a little more each time. Those men who follow this guideline are very surprised how good they feel in just a few weeks.
>
> Realistically, it may be four to eight weeks before you are 100% back to your presurgical stamina and strength.

can. Walking builds up your endurance, reduces risks for fatal blood clots and brings back that feeling of well-being and health. You should gradually build up the intensity, walking longer distances each day.

How soon can I get back into my regular exercise?

If you are an active person, you will need to gauge what you do by how your recovery progresses. Let your doctor guide you. We don't want you to strain or hurt yourself during the initial recovery phase, when your tissues aren't very strong. Whatever you do, move into it gradually. Don't sit back and avoid any activity and then suddenly jump in full speed. Rather, work into it slowly. Gradually build up your strength and skills.

How soon can I walk my dog?

This depends on the type of dog you have. If you are taking a tiny toy poodle out, any time you feel up to it is fine with me. On the other hand, if you want to walk—or be walked by—your rottweiler or Great Dane, I suggest you wait several weeks.

How soon after surgery will I be able to resume golf?

I usually encourage my golfing patients to keep active, and when they feel up to it, go out with the guys and just walk the course. Initially, you may only want to do a few short walking bursts and then ride a cart the rest of the way.

I don't want you to take full driving swings off the tee too soon. But when you're feeling stronger, I think it's reasonable to practice your chipping and putting. Several weeks after surgery you should be able to play without restrictions.

How soon can I start playing tennis or racquetball?

Tennis and racquetball require certain straining, so I ask that you hold off playing full speed until about four to six weeks from the day of your surgery. But until then, you should be able to go out and gently hit a few balls at about half speed. But remember, plain walking is the best exercise after surgery to get your strength and endurance back.

How quickly can I resume bicycle riding?

Bicycle riding is something you need to avoid until you really have recovered at six weeks or later after surgery. You should avoid putting pressure on your perineum during the initial recovery phase. This is the general area where your bladder and urethra have been surgically connected, and of course this is also what you sit on for bicycling.

When you do resume biking, do it slowly. You might find it more comfortable if you don't sit on a narrow, firm seat. The best seats are the no-nose seats (check out www.no-nose.com). A wider seat with more padding would make your transition back to cycling more pleasant.

What about using stair-steppers and the treadmill?

These activities you can start doing right away. Just be aware that you won't have the endurance you had before surgery.

What about weight lifting?

You should avoid strenuous weight lifting for a full six weeks from the time of surgery. Light arm exercises are okay until then.

How soon can I start bowling again?

Wait several weeks, depending on how good you feel. The bowling ball weighs more than I want you to carry until the incision is fully healed.

> *How soon after surgery will I be able to drive a car?*
>
> **?**
>
> You should not drive a car for at least two weeks after surgery, for two reasons.
>
> First, your incision is healing and may be tender. If you were driving and an emergency occurred or sudden braking was required, you may hesitate or be unable to perform at 100% because of pain or discomfort. You would be putting yourself and others at risk. It is generally accepted that after a major abdominal operation, you need a few weeks to recover enough to drive safely.
>
> Second, if you are involved in an accident and you just had a radical prostatectomy, even if it's not your fault, your legal position might look questionable.

How soon can I paint my house?

I usually suggest waiting three to four weeks before doing moderate work around the house, especially if much straining is involved. If you plan to stand on a ladder, then you should wait a full six weeks.

Can I work in my garden?

Yes, as long as you don't do any heavy lifting or straining. It is okay to bend over and do light gardening activities. Just take it easy and start slowly.

Travel

How soon can I be driven around town?

You can go out as soon as you are discharged from the hospital, as long as someone else drives you. The sooner you are up and around, the quicker your recovery will be.

Can I go as a passenger on a long trip?

Yes, if you must. Ideally, you should refrain from long trips for a few weeks. Long travel is okay only if at least every hour you get up out of your seat (or out of a car) and walk around to keep the blood moving through your veins. I also recommend that you wear support stockings.

How long after surgery should I wait before traveling?
If you're planning an elective vacation, I usually ask that you wait about four to six weeks to be sure you are well on your way to recovery. You can travel any time if you need to, but don't do any heavy lifting or straining. This means you can't carry your own luggage and should use all the help you can get.

Bathing

Can I shower or bathe after I go home?
Yes, there are no limits on showering or bathing. I prefer that you not take tub baths for a week or two. Avoid the potential strain of climbing in and out of a tub. Most men find it easier to shower for the first few weeks.

How soon can I swim after surgery?
I ask that you wait until the catheter comes out. By then, the incision will be fairly well healed, and you should be able to do light swimming. You should avoid strenuous swimming for about four to six weeks.

Can I use a hot tub, Jacuzzi or sauna after I get home?
You probably should avoid these for a few weeks until the incision has had a chance to heal and the catheter is out.

Support Stockings

Why do I need to wear the support stockings?
After surgery, the reduced blood flow through the veins and the reduced walking puts you at increased risk for developing blood clots for up to six to eight weeks after surgery. Blood clots in the legs can be painful, and they can also be quite dangerous if they break loose and move up to the lungs. Large blood clots can cause sudden death if they block large blood vessels. This is why we encourage you not only to walk frequently after surgery but also to

wear support stockings when you're just lying around. The stockings work by compressing the veins and reducing the odds of blood pooling in the veins.

How long should I wear support stockings after I go home?

Technically you are at risk for developing blood clots in the veins of the legs and pelvis for as long as six to eight weeks. With this in mind, I usually recommend that whenever you are going to be inactive for an extended period, like being a passenger on a long car or airplane trip, it is a good idea to wear support stockings. If you are active and walking quite a lot, then you do not have to wear them. If they don't drive you crazy, then I suggest wearing them for about six to eight weeks after surgery.

I wear them regularly (no, not the white ones) because I am on my feet for extended periods. Wearing them can increase your comfort, so keep them on even after the eight-week time if you feel you need to.

Diet

When will I be able to eat after surgery?

You should be able to eat anything you want after you get home. You may have a tendency toward constipation, so get plenty of fiber and bulk in your diet, and drink plenty of water and fluids.

Should I take iron supplements?

Taking iron supplements is probably a good idea, at least for the first few weeks after you leave the hospital. The supplements will provide plenty of iron to rebuild your blood counts. Iron can be constipating, so drink plenty of fluids and increase the fiber in your diet.

Are there any dietary restrictions after I go home?

There are no limits on what you can eat. You may be a little anemic, with a low blood count, but a balanced diet with some foods high in iron should be adequate.

What if I get constipated after I get home?
I usually recommend that you take some milk of magnesia or Dulocolax tablets as a gentle laxative. If your constipation is severe, talk with your doctor about medications such as Colace or Surfak, which can work to prevent constipation before it develops. It is important to drink plenty of fluids.

Incision

How long will it take the incision(s) to heal?
Most of the healing occurs within six weeks, but the incision(s) will continue to heal for six to twelve months.

Why does the incision(s) feel thick and hard?
This is your body's way of healing normally. As the tissues slowly heal, the thickening and firmness will gradually go away.

How will I know if I'm developing a skin infection in the incision?
Usually there will be increased tenderness, possibly redness and maybe even drainage of pus from the incision.

What can be done for an infection in the incision?
Usually opening up the incision where the infection is located will allow drainage and normal healing. Sometimes I'll start my patient on antibiotics if I'm really concerned. I may even pack some sterile gauze into the incision opening to help with drainage of infection. The open incision will heal naturally over time.

Can I do anything to help the incision(s) heal?
Keep the incision(s) out of the sun. Sun exposure can cause the delicate new skin tissues to become permanently tanned. After surgery, the incision will first be red. Then over a few months, it will gradually fade into normal skin color.

How are my insides different now after surgery?
You are missing your prostate gland and the adjacent seminal vesicles, as well as the lymph nodes that drain the prostate. The bladder is now attached

directly to the urethra, rather than to the prostate gland as it was before surgery. There are no other changes internally.

What if there continues to be pain where the intravenous line went into the skin?

This pain is common, but occasionally it can represent an infection or blockage of veins in the arm. Unless the infection spreads, it is easily treated with heat, ideally warm compresses. If it has quite a lot of redness and tenderness, then it may be an infection. You will probably need to be put on antibiotics, and you should watch the area closely.

How often do I have to be seen by my urologist for follow-up after surgery?

It is smart for you to see your urologist about seven to ten days after surgery to do a quick check of the incision. Then you will follow-up for removal of the catheter. You should then be seen again about four to six weeks later just to see how you are doing, review the pathology report and discuss long-term follow-up.

Do I need to see my primary-care doctor right away after surgery?

Not usually, unless you are having medical problems unrelated to the surgery that need attention. I suggest that you call and talk to your doctor or the nurse just to let them know you are home and doing well.

HORMONE THERAPY

24

Hormone therapy—one of the oldest known and most effective prostate cancer treatments—can be used as a main treatment for some men with prostate cancer or as a pretreatment to improve the effectiveness of another treatment. Hormone therapy can be used as a first-line treatment or for advanced cancer. Many new therapies, medications and variations have expanded the role of hormone therapy.

What is hormone therapy?

This is a treatment where the male hormones (called *androgens*) are eliminated from the body. The most common male hormone is *testosterone*, which is made primarily in the testicles. Hormone therapy is also called androgen blockade and anti-androgen therapy.

Why do you remove testosterone from the body?

We remove the hormone from the body during treatment because prostate cancer is *hormone-sensitive*. This means that testosterone stimulates prostate cancer's growth.

When the hormone is eliminated from the body, the cancer generally stops growing and may actually go into a dormant phase, like going into hibernation.

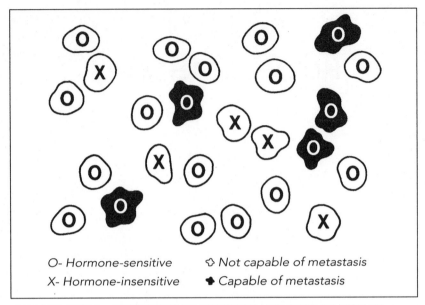

O- Hormone-sensitive   ✿ Not capable of metastasis
X- Hormone-insensitive   ✦ Capable of metastasis

CANCER CELLS—HORMONE SENSITIVITY AND RISK OF SPREAD.
Though the specific percentages vary from person to person and cancer to cancer, some of the prostate cancer cells are considered sensitive, while other cancer cells are referred to as hormone-insensitive and will not be affected by any change in testosterone levels. Likewise, some of the cancer cells are capable of spread, while others are thought to be incapable of spread, independent of their hormone sensitivity. This explains why cancers behave so variably and may not follow any set patterns or responses to treatment.

Similar to treatment of breast cancer, where women are given the opposite-sex hormone, men can be treated with female hormones or with other options that work to eliminate testosterone from the man's body.

Who is a candidate for hormone treatment?

Ideally, hormone therapy should be used for those men whose disease has shown signs of progression after radiation and/or surgery. Because so many men get good results from hormone therapy for several years, it is often used as the *primary treatment* in older men when we want to do something more than just follow the cancer but radiation or surgery is too much or is inappropriate.

What are other reasons to use hormone therapy?
One of the main reasons to use hormone therapy is for the treatment of wide-spread metastatic disease. If the cancer has spread to the lymph nodes or to the bones, hormone therapy is considered the correct treatment option. Hormone therapy may be used *before* or *during* radiation to improve results with high-grade and high-risk cancers.

Does hormone therapy work well for everyone?
When this treatment works, it works very well. But as with all treatments, everyone responds differently. Some men can go many years after hormone therapy with no evidence of any cancer growth. Most men will experience substantial cancer regression and shrinkage. For some, the cancer may remain dormant for many years, even ten years or more. Others may have good results for only a short period of time.

How can the cancer cells start to grow again?
Some cancers can learn to grow without the usual hormone stimulation. These cancers become hormone-insensitive.

In what situation is hormone therapy least likely to work?
The worst scenario is where the hormone treatment only seems to slow the cancer growth for a while, perhaps just a few months or years. This is seen with men who have a very aggressive cancer, often at an early age and with a very high PSA level. For these men, we're not sure hormone therapy will have much impact on the cancer's growth. For these few, it appears the most aggressive cancers are harder to treat and control.

Does hormone therapy actually cure the cancer?

No, not like radiation or surgery. Rather, the elimination of testosterone removes a major stimulant of the cancer's growth. Hormone therapy is an effective *control*, not a *cure*.

How can we tell which cancers will respond to hormone therapy and which won't?

At present we do not have any reliable way of testing to see who will and who won't benefit. It is thought that if you are a candidate for hormone therapy, you should be given a trial. If it works, and it usually does, then you have your answer.

Will hormone therapy prolong my life span?

We hope so and think so, but this is *not* guaranteed. Each person is different. For many men, hormone therapy offers many years of quality, comfortable life. For others, the cancer may be so aggressive that it may not respond to hormone treatments. If the cancer does respond, hormone therapy may only work for a few months rather than the expected years.

Will hormone treatment improve my quality of life?

For most men, we hope hormone therapy will keep the cancer from growing. There are potential side effects, however, that can possibly reduce the quality of your life.

What are the possible side effects of hormone therapy?

The most common side effect men complain of is hot flashes. These occur in 10% to 15% of men receiving hormone injections and a bit less after orchiectomy. (Injections and orchiectomy are explained later in this chapter.)

For most men, hot flashes seem to come and go. Then they may gradually become less frequent and less bothersome. For a few men, however, they can be quite overwhelming and disabling. Flashes can come on without warning and result in waves of heat and sweats. Fortunately for many men, the flashes tend to be self-limiting and slowly go away over time. Most men just put up with them.

TREATMENTS FOR HOT FLASHES

DES (Risks!)	Flutamide/Bicalutamide
Megace	Progesterone
Clonidine patch	Estrogen patch
Stop injections	

What causes hot flashes?
No one really understands how eliminating testosterone from your body brings on hot flashes.

What can be done to treat hot flashes?
Different men respond to different treatments. We have seen success with Clonidine patches, the hormone Megace every other day or daily for the first two weeks after each injection, Provera twice a day, estrogen patches once or twice a week and even low-dose estrogens (DES). DES and estrogens are explained later in this chapter.

What other side effects might occur?
Most men do well and are very happy and content with hormone therapy. Others may be bothered by any number of side effects from the elimination of testosterone from the body. Each person is different. You will only know how you tolerate the treatment once you have tried it. Potential side effects include fatigue, loss of energy, weight gain, loss of bone mass, loss of muscle mass, depression, emotional extremes (moodiness), problems with thinking processes and anemia.

I heard that some men have breast problems with hormones. Is this true?
Yes, breast tenderness and/or fullness does occur in a small percentage of men after starting hormone therapy. In many, the tenderness will eventually go away. Rarely, patients may require low-dose radiation or surgery to remove the enlarged or tender breast tissues.

Will hormone therapy affect my voice or behavior?
No. Hormone therapy will not affect your voice, outward appearance or behavior.

Will hormone therapy cause erectile dysfunction (make me impotent)?
Yes, it may very well remove your ability to have an erection. Or, it may possibly reduce the *quality* of the erections you have. Quite often, it will eliminate your desire and interest in sexual activity.

How will the effectiveness of hormone therapy be monitored?
If you have had an orchiectomy (castration), we know that your testosterone will drop to "castrate" levels, less than 20 ng/dl. If you are taking injections or other treatments, then you should have your testosterone level checked when you have your PSA checked to be sure your therapy is achieving a testosterone less than 20. If the testosterone is higher, then you may need to add on or change your treatment.

Though the PSA blood test is the best marker to follow and measure the impact of the treatment on the cancer, it is less helpful once you have initiated hormone therapy. Testosterone is needed for the cancer cells to grow and produce PSA. When testosterone is removed, the ability of the cancer cells to produce PSA is altered. Ideally, the PSA should drop to very low levels.

POTENTIAL SIDE EFFECTS OF HORMONE THERAPY

Hot flashes
Breast enlargement
Impotence
Breast tenderness
Reduced sex drive

Should I start the hormone treatments immediately?
Yes. Recent studies have shown an improved survival advantage to those men who started hormone therapy early as opposed to waiting. There are those who believe urologists should wait as long as possible until there are definite symptoms of the cancer spreading before hormone treatment is started. I disagree with this delaying approach. I believe in early treatment as soon as the advanced disease is identified. I think this approach provides the best long-term results.

How is this done?

There are several ways of undergoing hormone therapy today. For years, men were simply given the female hormone estrogen (DES) as a once-a-day pill. This worked well to stop the cancer's growth. Unfortunately, estrogen has serious potential side effects in men, which are discussed below.

Because of these life-threatening side effects, the use of estrogen has fallen out of favor. Instead, we now tend to remove the testicles (source of testosterone) surgically (orchiectomy). Or we may give an injection of an artificial hormone that tricks the body into stopping testosterone production (LHRH therapy). Both treatments are equally effective in decreasing male hormone levels in the body.

OPTIONS FOR HORMONE THERAPY

Antiandrogen (Casodex, Eulexin, Nilandron)
Estrogen (DES)
LHRH Analog (Lupron, Zoladex, Trelstar, Eligard or Viadur)
LHRH Antagonist (Abarelix)
Orchiectomy (removal of testicles)

DES (Diethylstilbestrol)

What is DES?

Diethylstilbestrol, called *DES* for short, is a type of estrogen or female hormone.

Why isn't DES used anymore?

Most doctors stopped using DES as a primary treatment several years ago when safer alternative treatments became available. DES has been associated with heart attacks, strokes and fatal blood clots. DES may be used in selected men with advanced disease, often with blood thinners to prevent complications.

How long does it take for DES to drop the testosterone levels?

It can take 30 to 60 days after starting DES therapy for testosterone levels to reach their lowest level.

What if I'm already on DES and have had no problems?
If you've been on DES for a few years, you'll probably continue to do well. There is a risk of developing heart problems, strokes or blood clots. I recently had an elderly patient who had been maintained on DES for over ten years, doing well without any side effects. I explained my concerns and his options, and he chose to continue with DES therapy.

What are the advantages of DES therapy?
DES is fairly inexpensive ($10 to $20 per month) and easy to take, just one pill each day.

Orchiectomy

What is an orchiectomy?
Surgical removal of the testicles, also called *castration*.

Is removal of the testicles an effective treatment?
Yes, this results in a very rapid and effective drop in the testosterone level to almost zero. This treatment is *permanent*. You don't have to worry about testosterone levels sneaking back up, and you don't have to worry about daily pills or monthly injections.

Orchiectomy is the gold standard against which all other hormone treatments are measured. Some claim to be as good. None are better.

Why would a man care about keeping his testicles if this is the best treatment?
Some men simply don't want or like the idea of having their testicles removed when there is a less traumatic option. It is an emotional issue. It has to do with one's self-image. In talking with patients about this option, I explain that they get to keep their scrotum intact and that we only remove the testicles from within the scrotum. Based on this knowledge, some men then decide to go ahead with this procedure.

How quickly does the operation lower my testosterone levels?
The testosterone level drops rapidly down to zero, within three to twelve hours. Men with pain from cancer in the bone may experience disappearance of the pain within a few days or less! I had one patient who was riddled with cancer. He noted a dramatic improvement and almost total elimination of bone pain the next day.

How is an orchiectomy done?
This is performed as an outpatient procedure where you go into a hospital or outpatient facility, have the operation and go home a few hours later.

Under anesthesia, the testicles are removed through a small incision in the front of the scrotum. Each testicle is separated from surrounding attachments. The blood vessels are then clamped and tied off with suture material. Some prefer a subcapsular orchiectomy where the testosterone-producing tissues are removed, leaving the outer shell of the testicle intact.

The testicles are removed and sent to pathology to be analyzed for cancer, even though cancer in the testicles is extremely rare.

Who actually does the surgery?
Usually done by a urologist, the procedure can easily be done by a general surgeon if no urologist is available. It is considered a relatively easy operation to perform.

What are the main risks of this surgery?
Complications after an orchiectomy are quite rare. The two concerns following this operation are infection and bleeding. These risks definitely shouldn't keep you from having the operation. You should not be alarmed if you have a little swelling or some bruising, which is common.

If you notice increased redness, swelling or pain, or if the incision starts to ooze pus-like drainage, you need to inform your doctor and be seen right away. You may have developed an infection of the incision. Your doctor will most likely start you on antibiotics, or he or she might open the incision slightly to allow drainage. Infections are rare because of the good blood supply to the scrotal skin.

The other problem is potentially more serious but also rare—serious bleeding. If a small blood vessel starts to bleed after the surgery, the scrotum can swell up rapidly, turn purple and look like a large eggplant. This is a *true emergency*. It requires immediate surgical exploration under anesthesia to identify and tie off the bleeding blood vessels and to drain out the blood built up in the scrotum.

What type of anesthesia will I need?

There are two basic types of anesthesia that can be used for this operation. The most common is general anesthesia where you are put to sleep for the entire operation. The second most common is called a *MAC* (*monitored anesthesia care*), where the anesthesiologist gives you a sedative through your veins. The sedative puts you out long enough to allow the surgeon to inject a long-acting numbing anesthetic solution into the tissues. You would then return to a partially sedated state. You won't feel anything during the rest of the operation.

In a few men, I have even performed the orchiectomy under a local anesthetic with no sedation at all. The choice is up to you. Sometimes your general health may suggest that one anesthesia may be safer than another for you. Talk with the anesthesiologist.

Will I need to have stitches removed?

Most doctors use absorbable stitches, so you should not need to have any removed. They dissolve on their own. Occasionally the skin edges may open up. This is quite common and will usually heal quickly on its own. I recommend that you keep the incision clean and dry, washing with a diluted

Will there be pain after an orchiectomy?

There is usually no pain, but some men complain of an ache or soreness for a few days. Most are surprised how easy it is and how good they feel afterward. There can be some swelling of tissues or even a little bruising, but this isn't usually a problem.

hydrogen-peroxide solution once or twice a day. You may want to use an antibiotic ointment such as Bacitracin or the equivalent once or twice a day.

What happens after I go home?

To make your recovery easier, it is best to avoid heavy lifting and straining for the first week or two. You should apply ice packs to the scrotum every hour or so for the first 48 hours to keep the swelling down. Be careful to apply the ice over a layer of clothing and not directly to the skin, as this can cause injury.

When can I shower?

Anytime you wish is okay. I recommend not taking a tub bath until the incision is totally healed, usually about a week or two after surgery.

When can I drive?

If you are not taking any pain medications you should be able to drive within a few days. Ask your doctor.

Injection Therapy

What kind of medication will block testosterone production?

The medication is called an *LHRH injection*. It is basically a copy of a naturally occurring hormone in the body that actually stimulates the production of testosterone. Another type actually blocks testosterone production.

How do these injections work?

LHRH medication stimulates the brain to produce a short burst of testosterone for about two weeks. Your body interprets this burst as having *too much* testosterone. Your brain, sensing too much testosterone, essentially *shuts down* testosterone production. In about 85% of men, this results in the same low level of hormone in the body as if the testicles had been removed. To maintain the benefits of these injections, you should continue them for the rest of your life. The removal of testosterone stimulates normal programmed cell death (apoptosis) in cancer cells. This results in the dying of cancer cells that need the testosterone to grow.

Could the flare-up of the hormone right after the start of the shots
cause any problems?

This is a rare but potentially serious problem if the cancer has already spread alongside the spinal cord in the backbone. If there is prostate cancer in the spine, then a bone scan may show the location. Only a CT scan or MRI would show that it may be squeezing the spinal cord. It is not standard procedure to order these tests in most circumstances unless we are suspicious.

The cancer may possibly increase in size during the flare-up of testosterone levels, which can squeeze and damage the spinal cord. Though rare, this could cause you to become paralyzed.

What are the advantages of LHRH shots?

You get to keep your testicles and still receive an effective treatment to drop your testosterone level. Later, if you have side effects, such as the hot flashes mentioned earlier, and you are intolerant of the treatments, then you could choose to have the orchiectomy. These injections also work if you opt for intermittent therapy (explained later in this chapter).

Are the various types of hormone shots the same?

They effectively do the same thing but are slightly different variations on the same theme. From a medical point of view, they are equally effective and are as effective as removal of the testicles in decreasing testosterone. There is another medication, Abarelix, that, instead of stimulating the hormone to drop testosterone, actually works to block testosterone production. This approach eliminates the flare of testosterone, though there are some risks and side effects that can be of concern. Degarelix is a new drug just approved.

What are the hormone medications?

There are several kinds of LHRH analog medications available: Lupron (leuprolide acetate), Zoladex (goserelin acetate implant), Trelstar (triptorelin pamoate), Eligard (leuprolide acetate) and Vantas (histrelin implant). They are similar and work the same way to cause a drop in testosterone.

How are the injections given?

Lupron, Trelstar and Eligard are given as an injection into the muscle of one of the buttocks. Many doctors will alternate from one side to the other, as they make subsequent injections. Degarelix is given subcutaneously.

Zoladex is a pellet that is injected into the tissue just under the surface of the skin, usually given somewhere on the upper abdominal wall. This is considered a good location, because this area has fewer nerves and a good blood supply. This injection usually first requires administration of a tiny amount of local anesthetic to numb the skin before the pellet is inserted. Then the pellet is inserted through a tiny nick in the skin made with the injection needle. Some doctors prefer to give the injection without first numbing the skin.

One-, three-, and four-month versions are available for many of these medications. Once you have established that you tolerate this treatment, you may opt to receive the medication in longer intervals. There is even a once-a-year subcutaneous implant (Vantas) that is placed just under the skin of the arm.

How long does the treatment last?

If you choose hormone shots, you will need to continue them for the rest of your life. You can always switch from shots to the surgery, and then of course the shots would no longer be necessary. Occasionally with very advanced disease, we stop the shots when we try other treatments.

?

What if I'm late getting a treatment?

The benefit of injections is that they do not need to be given exactly on a set date. Being a little early or late shouldn't really make a difference. On an occasional basis, such fluctuations probably won't cause any problems, but I ask patients to stick to the schedule as closely as possible.

What do the shots cost?
Prices vary but in general are several hundred dollars each month. These costs are usually covered by insurance, HMOs and Medicare. You may be responsible for a small portion for your co-pay.

What if I miss a treatment?
Then you may have some return of male hormone to your system. Some experts suggest that you have some flexibility. In the big scheme of things, it probably won't be a problem. It's not a good idea to miss entire treatments regularly.

What is the goal of these medications?
The goal is to drop the testosterone level to 20 ng/dl or less. In about one out of five or six men, the testosterone level will be higher than 20, putting you at risk for failure of this treatment. When the testosterone level remains higher than 20, it is smart to add an antiandrogen.

Total Androgen Blockade

Do these hormone therapies eliminate all of the male hormone?
No, a small amount of the male hormones (*androgens*) are secreted by the *adrenal glands*, located on top of the kidneys. There is much debate whether or not this remaining male hormone plays a role in cancer-treatment failures. Some experts believe that in addition to the injections of LHRH analog, or removal of the testicles, you should also take another medicine daily called an *antiandrogen*. These drugs are flutamide (Eulexin), bicalutamide (Casodex) or Nilutamide (Nilandron). Eulexin must be taken three times a day, Casodex just once a day and Nilandron, once a day.

How do antiandrogens work?
Antiandrogens block the cancer cells' ability to absorb testosterone or DHT, producing what is called *total* or *complete androgen blockade*. Blocking these hormones prevents the cancer cells' stimulation and growth. There are experts who believe the combination of LHRH injections and antiandrogens keep the cancer in check longer than monthly injections alone.

> How long do I have to take antiandrogens?
>
> **?**
>
> Antiandrogens are intended to be taken for the rest of your life. If you're taking antiandrogens and the cancer starts to come back (the PSA starts to rise again), the medication may be stopped to see if you have a drop in your PSA levels. This is called the *antiandrogen withdrawal response (AAWR)*. Why this occurs, no one really knows. It does not occur in everyone. This drop in PSA can be for a short time or last many months or more.

Can I take antiandrogens at a later time if there's a concern the cancer is growing?

If you are not on antiandrogens and at some point your PSA level starts to go up, then antiandrogens can always be added to your treatment, usually with good results. Again, if your testosterone level does not drop to castrate levels with the LHRH injections alone, then it would be better to start antiandrogens sooner.

What do Casodex, Eulexin or Nilandron cost?

These hormones cost from $200 to $350 per month. While this cost can be a financial burden for some men, it is usually covered by insurance.

What are the side effects of Casodex, Eulexin or Nilandron?

The primary significant side effect of Eulexin is diarrhea. This can be quite significant and very upsetting if it is severe or prolonged. If you start antiandrogens and get diarrhea, we usually reduce the dose.

If diarrhea is still a problem, we will stop the Eulexin altogether to see if it is really the culprit or if you just have a touch of intestinal flu. Even if the diarrhea goes away, we will restart the medication slowly and gradually build back up to a full dose, three times each day.

If you have a history of liver disease you may need to be careful, as the antiandrogens can increase liver damage, but this is rare. If we have any questions, we will monitor you with blood tests to make sure there is no liver damage.

Nilandron is not used very often because of an uncommon problem with reduced night vision in changing light in 12% of men.

Intermittent Therapy

What is intermittent therapy?
This is where we start and stop the hormone therapy. Specifically, you will start hormone therapy, then stop it when your PSA drops to its lowest level and stabilizes. At this point we hope your side effects go away. Hormone therapy would be restarted when the PSA level starts to climb again. Therapy would be continued until the PSA again drops back down, and the cycle is repeated. Usually you will be on or off therapy for six months to a year or more, depending on your response and how well you tolerate the treatment.

This pattern of on-and-off hormone therapy would be less expensive than continuous therapy. If you are bothered by hot flashes or impotence or any of the other side effects, intermittent therapy might give you occasional breaks with a return to normal life, and improved quality of life.

Use of Hormones Before Surgery or Radiation

Why does my doctor want me to take hormone shots before I have surgery?
The hope is that by using hormone shots for two to eight months before surgery, the size of the prostate may be reduced and make the surgery easier to perform. Though it doesn't work for everyone, many men with large prostates can have a significant reduction in prostate size with a few months of hormone therapy. There is still debate about whether it really makes a difference.

Can taking hormone shots make the cancer shrink?
This was originally the idea when hormone therapy was given before surgery. There are a large number of studies comparing men who had hormone shots before surgery with men who didn't. Most researchers feel that if it does shrink the cancer, it is only in a small percentage of those men having prostate surgery. In my experience, the hormone pretreatment, called *neoadjuvant therapy*, really hasn't made much of a difference.

What is the reason not to try the hormone shots before surgery?
The main concern expressed by my patients is the fear of unpleasant side effects, such as impotence and hot flashes.

Can hormone shots be used to keep the cancer from spreading if I can't have surgery or radiation for several months?
Yes, hormone therapy may work to prevent continued cancer growth. If the cancer has already grown outside the prostate, hormone therapy will probably not change this.

If my PSA level falls dramatically after hormone shots, do I have to go ahead with surgery?
Yes. Hormone therapy isn't a long-term cure. It's a short-term control. Under the influence of hormone therapy, it is common to see the PSA level drop dramatically. This does not mean the cancer has gone away, but rather that the ability to secrete the PSA substance is reduced. In other words, the cancer is still there.

Would it help to take hormone shots before radiation?
In selected men with large prostates or aggressive cancer, hormone therapy before treatment appears to improve the effectiveness of the radiation.

Is there any reason to stay on hormone shots even after radiation?
Yes, if the cancer is high-grade or large and is thought to be potentially very aggressive, then staying on hormone therapy may provide better long-term cure rates than radiation alone.

Can any other problems occur with long-term hormone therapy?
Anemia is commonly seen with prostate cancer patients, and is associated with androgen deprivation. It is important to monitor your blood count initially and during hormone therapy. There are a number of treatment options, including medications that can stimulate your body to increase the blood count. If the anemia is significant, some men have to stop the hormone therapy for a period of time (intermittent hormone therapy).

Option	Cost	Type of Treatment	Side Effects	Benefits
DES	$30/Month Lifetime	Daily Pill	High-Dose Risks: Heart Attack Stroke Blood Clots	Inexpensive, Effective
Orchiec-tomy	$2500+ One-Time	Outpatient Surgery	Hot Flashes Breast En-largement	Quick, Single Treatment Rapid Drop in Hormones Overall Less Expensive
Lupron/ Zoladex/ Trelstar/ Eligard/ Vantas/ Degarelix	$400–$500/Month Lifetime	Injections	Hot flashes Breast Tenderness	Avoid Surgery
Casodex/ Eulexin/ Nilandron	$230–$320/Month Lifetime	Daily pills	Diarrhea, Impaired Night Vi-sion(12%)	May Prolong Survival

Osteoporosis is often seen with hormone therapy, because testosterone, which is eliminated, helps stimulate bone growth. The longer you are on hormone therapy, the higher your risks for bone problems and even fractures. The bones are in a constant state of growth and resorption, so this reduction in bone growth can result in weakening of the bones. Rarely do men describe bone pain in their hands or feet after starting hormone therapy. This osteoporosis can be treated with a graduated exercise program, which can stimulate bone growth, as well as with medications called bisphosphonates that slow bone resorption. This is supplemented with calcium and synthetic vitamin D and fluoride, which strengthen the bones further.

Some men also describe fatigue and decreased muscle mass.

How does prostate metastasis weaken bones?

To understand the answer, you need to know how bone structure is normally maintained. Bone is an active, living tissue. In the normal bone, there is a balance between bone-building cells (osteoblasts) and bone-destroying cells (osteoclasts). The bone offers a fertile environment for prostate cancer to grow. When prostate cancer cells spread to the bone, they alter the normal balance, and stimulate abnormal bone growth in some areas, and abnormal bone weakening in others. This results in a weakening of the bones. This is like building a brick wall—it's not the total number of bricks, but how they are put together that gives the wall its strength or weakness.

What are bisphosphonates?

They are a category of medications that strengthen weakened bones from osteoporosis or when cancer has spread to the bone. Bisphophonates can reduce pain from cancer in the bone. One such drug is Zometa.

How is zoledronic acid given?

Zoledronic acid (Zometa) is given intravenously over 15 minutes every three weeks. This is continued as long as there is risk for bone weakening or bone pain. It is important to drink plenty of fluids, and monitor your kidney function before the medication is given. Many people experience flu-like symptoms afterward for a short time. A rare side effect is a serious jaw problem, so if you have any dental, gum or jaw problems, you need to tell your doctors as they may have to avoid Zometa.

CRYOTHERAPY AND HIFU—
FREEZING AND HEATING
THE PROSTATE

25

B oth cryotherapy and HIFU work through opposite ways to achieve the same goal: to kill prostate cancer cells. Each has advantages and disadvantages, but they are similar in techniques, side effects and indications. At the present time, they both look very promising and offer more choices for initial treatment of prostate cancer or when radiation has failed.

Cryotherapy

Cryotherapy can be a viable treatment for some men with prostate cancer when performed by experienced surgeons. Though not available in many parts of the country, certain centers and urologists have the experience and a very promising track record with cryotherapy, both for initial treatment for prostate cancer and also for treatment when other options fail.

What is cryotherapy?
This is the controlled freezing of the prostate gland for cancer treatment, the intention being to kill the cancer cells.

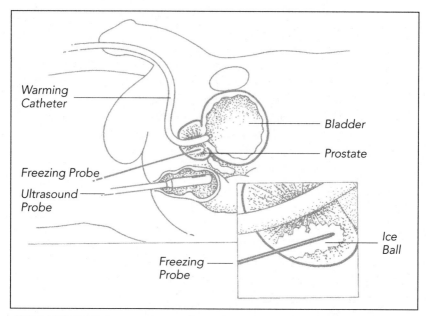

CRYOSURGERY. Prostate tissue is frozen by probes inserted directly into the prostate. This creates an ice ball of prostate tissue, killing the cancer cells. A catheter placed in the urethra circulates a solution to keep it warm during the procedure. An ultrasound probe is used to be sure that the rectal wall is not frozen.

Is cryotherapy the same as cryosurgery?

Yes, they refer to the same treatment. *Cryosurgical ablation* and *targeted cryoablation* mean the same thing.

What is the role for cryosurgery?

This is a developing technique in which the prostate tissue is *frozen*. The purpose is to kill the cancer cells. The relative simplicity, reduced costs, ease and quickness of cryosurgery make it potentially a better treatment than prostatectomy or lengthy radiation treatments. At this point, we don't know if cryotherapy will be effective as a long-term treatment for prostate cancer.

How is cryosurgery performed?

Cryosurgery is performed under anesthesia. Special probes are placed throughout the prostate. Their positions are confirmed with rectal ultrasound. Liquid nitrogen or Argon gas is circulated through the probes, freezing the tissue of

When is cryotherapy best?

It may be good as an option *after* or *instead* of radiation treatment. As with all evolving techniques, the final answer still is not yet known. Even experts who are regularly doing this procedure are not sure of the role for cryosurgery in the future. In time, cryotherapy may be used on a large number of men with prostate cancer. Then perhaps we'll know if this is another great idea that just didn't work or if it is the great answer we've been waiting for.

the prostate. A rectal ultrasound probe is used to monitor the freezing and to let the surgeon know when enough tissue has been treated.

The goal is to create an ice ball big enough to kill the cancer. According to supporters of this technique, there is no damage to the adjacent bladder or to the rectal wall, which lies just behind the prostate.

The long-term results are promising. There are concerns that some cancer cells may escape being frozen, and other cells may be outside the prostate and would not be treated. Others have concerns over side effects. Preliminary results with newer techniques in experienced hands look promising.

Does cryotherapy also freeze the urethra?

A catheter is placed in the urethra to circulate a warming solution that protects the urethra from freezing during treatment.

Does cryosurgery work with big prostates?

Not really. It works best when the prostate gland is measured with ultrasound to be about 40 grams or less in size.

What can be done if I've been told that I have a large prostate, but I want cryotherapy?

You could try to shrink the gland with three to eight months of total hormone blockade, using both the monthly shots and the antiandrogens. You would then need ultrasound reevaluation to confirm that the prostate is small enough to be effectively treated by cryotherapy.

Can I have cryotherapy if I've already had a TURP?

Yes, but it is harder to perform with less precise freezing. Cryosurgery is best done in prostates that have not had previous surgery.

What are the most common side effects of cryotherapy?

The treatment can cause quite a lot of irritation to the bladder or urethra, resulting in many symptoms such as frequent urination with little warning, burning, blood, pain with urination and similar symptoms of irritation to the rectal wall. Almost half of men who have cryotherapy complain of some degree of penile or scrotal swelling. This is usually temporary.

What else can cause problems after cryotherapy?

Some men develop scars in the urethra, while others can have trouble urinating, requiring a catheter. Fortunately, these risks are relatively uncommon.

Can I become incontinent after cryosurgery?

This is relatively rare and shouldn't be a problem after cryosurgery.

Are there any other serious complications from cryotherapy?

In addition to the irritation symptoms, the two main risks are the potential formation of an abnormal connection between the urethra and rectum, called a *fistula*, and possible incomplete treatment of the cancer.

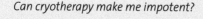

?

Can cryotherapy make me impotent?

Yes. Up to 80% or more of men who undergo cryotherapy complain of impotence afterward. The risk of impotence depends on how aggressively the surgeon freezes the prostate tissues. Remember, the goal is to kill cancer cells.

HIFU (High Intensity Focused Ultrasound)

What is HIFU?

HIFU is a new and exciting technique that uses proven concepts of high-energy heat for the treatment of prostate cancer.

Where else was this technology used?

A variation of the HIFU concept has been used successfully to treat non-cancerous prostate enlargement.

How does HIFU work?

High-energy ultrasound waves are focused through a rectal probe into the prostate. This ultrasound energy is then directed into the prostate under real-time guidance. Next, this energy is rapidly converted into heat within the meat of the prostate, and thus it effectively "cooks" the prostate tissue, killing the cancer cells.

Is this done in the office?

No, because of the technique and time required, HIFU is performed under an anesthesia as an outpatient.

How long does HIFU take?

The actual procedure takes about one to three hours. This is because on average 400 to 600 pulses of microwave energy are focused into the prostate. Plus, some time is needed setting up and getting you ready as well as recovery time afterward.

When is HIFU an option to consider?

HIFU appears to be used primarily as an initial therapy for localized prostate cancer or to treat the prostate for rising PSA after radiation (radiation failure).

What about risks for incontinence and ED (erectile dysfunction, also called impotence) after HIFU?

Early results show low rates of ED and incontinence. Again, this procedure is very operator dependent so be sure to seek out an experienced doctor if you opt for HIFU.

Who should perform HIFU?

Only doctors with special training and experience should perform HIFU. As with any procedure, you should seek doctors who have the highest level of experience. Using a skilled doctor will provide better chances for success with fewer side effects or complications.

What is MRgFUS?

This is the use of MRI for magnetic resonance–guided therapy, as compared with ultrasound guidance.

What side effects do you expect after HIFU?

Because the prostate tissue is heated so rapidly and dies, you might see side effects of inflammation, swelling and irritation similar to cryotherapy. These irritative symptoms usually pass with time and resolution of the inflammation and swelling of the prostate. Some men may urinate better with alpha-blockers and anti-inflammation medications.

Do I need a catheter afterwards?

Yes, you will need a Foley catheter for seven to ten days to allow your bladder to drain while most of the prostate swelling resolves.

COMPLEMENTARY, INTEGRATIVE AND ALTERNATIVE TREATMENTS

26

There has been almost a feeding frenzy over the past few years regarding nontraditional treatments for almost every complaint or disease—including prostate cancer. Much of this interest relates to our continued fascination with Eastern and herbal therapies as well as our desire to find the "magic" pill that will offer a cure with no risks. Recently, many traditional physicians and institutions have realized and accepted that there may be a valid role for some of these alternatives in the treatment of prostate-cancer patients.

Unfortunately, many of these new treatments are without any scientific support or research. And some may even be dangerous. It is essential for you to understand everything you can about these products before you agree to take them.

Do the terms "nutritional," "herbal," "nontraditional," and "alternative" all mean the same thing?

Not exactly. They all suggest treatments that do not use standard surgery, radiation, hormone blockade or chemotherapy. It is very important to understand the role of these treatment options. Many leading experts refer to these treatment choices as *complementary* or *integrative*.

Do some of these complementary or integrative options really work?

I personally believe in many of the complementary and integrative approaches, but I have serious concerns about many of the alternative options—options that are still unproven, yet are heavily promoted as if they are valid treatments. And while you wait to see if some herbal concoction works, the commercial promoters have taken your money. And then what if it doesn't work as claimed? You're left struggling to salvage a potentially serious and dangerous prostate-cancer situation. I hear all the time of herbs and treatments taken off the market because of serious side effects—problems the proponents or manufacturers didn't mention.

Complementary means that the new treatment is intended to be used *in addition* to the standard proven treatment option—to complement what we already know to work.

Integrative means that the treatments are designed to work *together*—a blending of the best of both traditional and nontraditional treatment options.

Alternative suggests that the treatment is to be used *instead of* known and accepted treatments.

Isn't a natural approach always better than radiation, surgery or chemotherapy for prostate cancer?

Not usually. "Natural" simply means derived from the Earth, its plants or animals. Generally speaking, natural products are not better for you just because they are natural. Consider anthrax, botulism and plague—all natural but not things you'd want to have.

With all the hype and claims, how do we know what is reasonable to follow and what may just be sales propaganda?

That's a tough question. In general, I suggest that you remain skeptical of all claims until you've seen or heard them from a number of sources, not just the promoter selling the product. I like to subscribe to a number of reputable

Beware of testimonial-style marketing, where a small number of men and women claim to have had a "miraculous" recovery with a treatment.

newsletters, such as the *Johns Hopkins Medical Letter: Health After 50*, the *Mayo Clinic Health Letter*, the *Harvard Health Letter* or the *University of California at Berkeley Wellness Letter*. In addition, my favorite is Dr. Charles Myers's *Prostate Forum* newsletter, which focuses on dietary and nutritional aspects of prostate cancer, and the *Tufts University Health & Nutrition Letter*. (See chapter 39 for information on support groups and resources.)

Feel free to do health research on the Internet, but do so with some skepticism. As the men's health expert for WebMD for more than five years, I am naturally biased and think WebMD and similar education sites are a great and reliable resource for accurate information. Note if most of the Internet websites are for commercial sales or are informational. A valid product or treatment will have plenty of studies to back up any claims. Be wary of non-U.S. or third world studies—they often are paid for by the company promoting the product. Also watch out for sites promoting opinion as fact.

What kinds of things should I watch out for if I'm considering alternative treatments?

Be very careful if you hear claims that "organized medicine" is trying to "bury" or "ignore" a particular product so that doctors can continue to "profit off of illness." This claim may be followed by something like, "And by the way, you can buy our magic pills direct for only $49.95 a month." Whose best interest is really at stake here?

I have yet to meet a doctor who would ignore any proven treatment that would help his or her patient.

Some basic guidelines apply to the search for a doctor or a treatment, no matter who the provider is. First and foremost, what kind of training did that person receive? I knew of one health-care provider who had only taken a few weekend courses, yet claimed he had extensive training and experience in the field.

Beware of testimonial-style marketing, where a small number of men and women claim to have had a "miraculous" recovery with a treatment.

Are there any problems with following an alternative or unproven treatment?

Yes, there could be serious consequences. Be aware that there are two potential risks associated with unproven treatments. First, the treatment may not work and the cancer might continue to grow. If you are fortunate enough to be diagnosed when the cancer is still confined to the prostate gland, be wary that delaying standard treatments (and reliance on unproven alternatives) may allow the cancer to progress beyond the capsule, reducing the chances for cure later on with the more traditional treatments. The second and perhaps more worrisome problem is that the alternative treatment itself may actually be dangerous and cause you harm. Some herbs may increase risks of dangerous blood clots. Some studies have shown that certain vitamins may have harmful effects at higher doses.

Overall, the most common problem I've seen is that pursuing an alternative treatment can result in significant delays in obtaining an effective and proven treatment. Years ago, I remember a young man who was diagnosed with cancer, who decided to fly to Switzerland for oxygen injections, certain that they would cure him. Many months later, when he finally returned and requested to go ahead with treatments we had discussed, the cancer had progressed and he was no longer able to have one of the curative options.

The key is to integrate the treatment options. If you are young and have a significant cancer, and you want to follow a strict diet, then fine—do it AND have the surgery or radiation. Get the best of all treatment options to give you the maximum chance for a normal and healthy life.

If it looks easy, with results almost *too good to be true*, it usually is. If it is very expensive, beware. Many of these treatments require cash up front. This should make you very suspicious.

Watch out if this elaborate and expensive treatment is completed in just a weekend, especially if it is in a country with few limitations on unproven treatments.

More and more of my patients follow both traditional and alternative approaches to treating their prostate cancer. In my experience, this is almost always beneficial. However, I ask patients to let me know what they are doing so I will know how to deal with complications that may appear. Recently, after an uneventful radical prostatectomy, Jerome began to take herbal supplements that a friend at the nutrition store had recommended to hasten his recovery. Within 48 hours, Jerome began to bleed unexpectedly. Only after extensive tests and evaluations by several specialists did Jerome tell me he had been taking supplemental herbs. When we researched them, we discovered they were blood thinners and were causing the bleeding. Jerome was surprised to find that anything "natural" could have a negative effect on his health. Even "natural" remedies and therapies must be evaluated for their potential benefits or side effects.

Are there any herbs that can be dangerous?

Yes, a week doesn't go by that we don't learn from the newspapers of an unexpected and dangerous side effect of an herb that we all believed to be safe. Some herbs can cause severe liver damage, while others can thin the blood, leading to unexpected and serious bleeding during surgery. Some have been shown to reduce or increase the effectiveness of prescribed medications, which can be very hazardous. Recently, a few have actually been taken off the store shelves because of serious complications and death.

What about alternative therapy clinics that advertise such high cure rates?

Over the many years of my practice, I have had patients who have spent up to $30,000 or delayed their treatments by a year to follow what they were led to believe to be a nontraditional cure. Every single one of them had absolutely no success from these "mystery" treatments. I am worried that some of these patients may have actually ended up with worse problems because of the delays. Watch out for the doctor (and yes, M.D.'s too!) who claims to have a secret formula or treatment that (1) No one else has and (2) The rest of medicine doesn't want you to know about. These are two warning signs that you are about to be taken for a very expensive ride.

INCONTINENCE—
A POTENTIAL RISK

27

U rinary incontinence is the *involuntary* loss of urine. In other words, it is leaking urine when you don't know that you are or when you are trying not to. This condition can be a temporary or permanent side effect of treatment for prostate cancer, and it can be a major quality-of-life issue.

Under normal conditions, what keeps a man from leaking urine?
The key to bladder control is a combination of the circular muscle fibers at the bladder neck and the sphincter muscles located in the pelvic floor, beneath the bladder, surrounding the urethra. This muscle combination works to close off the urethra and prevent leakage of urine from the bladder.

Why do some men become incontinent of urine after a radical prostatectomy?
When the prostate is removed from the base of the bladder, damage can occur to the urinary sphincter that gives the man a mechanism for holding in urine naturally. This damage can result in incontinence. There are various surgical techniques for operating on this anatomy during a prostatectomy, but the potential danger of tissue and muscle damage is ever present.

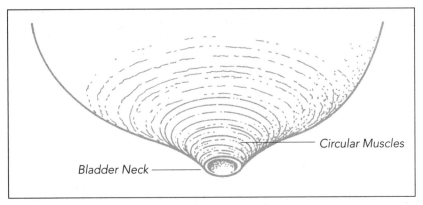

BLADDER NECK. Circular muscles of the bladder neck squeeze together to keep urine from leaking. These can be damaged during surgery or radiation, resulting in urinary incontinence.

Fine-tuned techniques and preservation of the tissues and nerves during prostatectomy have improved urinary control for most men.

What can I do to reduce the time I will leak after the catheter comes out?
Eventually, many men can relearn how to use the muscles damaged during surgery. I strongly encourage all my patients to begin *Kegel exercises* even before surgery.

What is a Kegel exercise?
It is simply an exercise to strengthen the pelvic muscles. This group of muscles can be exercised and trained to be stronger. This is the reason we encourage Kegel exercise for men who will undergo radical prostatectomy. After surgery, while the catheter is in place, it's important for you to continue working the pelvic muscles. I have had patients tell me that when they stop the exercises, they notice a dramatic increase in the amount of incontinence they have.

How do I do Kegel exercises?
You probably already do this exercise unknowingly. When you are urinating and suddenly stop midstream—that's the Kegel exercise! If you are standing in a public place and suddenly feel the urge to pass gas, and you "snug up"

the muscles to hold it in, that too is a Kegel exercise. I would best describe it as a *tightening of the pelvic muscles.*

Or—imagine that you are standing on top of a hill, naked, with a $1,000 bill tucked between the cheeks of your buttocks. You are not able to use your hands, but you need to hold onto the bill during high, gusty winds. That squeezing of your buttocks, pulling up internally and tightening down with your pelvic muscles, is a Kegel exercise.

Will people around me know I am doing the exercises?
If you are doing them correctly, no.

How often should I do the Kegel exercises?
You need to do them regularly, not just when you think of it. I suggest at least every hour for five minutes. When the catheter is removed, you should be doing the exercises at least 20 times a day. It is important that you don't just tighten up and then let go. Rather, tighten up and then hold it, then let go and repeat. Don't just do it as an exercise. Before surgery and after the catheter comes out, practice stopping midstream when you urinate. Hold it and then restart forcefully. This should help build up and restore the muscle tone.

How long should I continue to do the Kegel exercises?
You should continue to do these exercises as long as you have a problem with urinary leakage. This could be a few days to a few months. Rarely, some men may have to do them forever.

How long can I expect to leak urine after surgery?

?

There is no way to predict who will leak and who will not, or for how long. Some men note they never leaked after the catheter came out, while most describe a few weeks to a few months or more of continued leakage. A few patients have complained of continued leakage for more than a year before it stopped. A small percentage of men will have continued leaking *permanently.* Fortunately, this severe leaking is fairly rare.

If the leakage goes on for a very long time, does that mean it will never stop?

No. Some of my patients have reported continued leakage to some degree for many months before everything "dried up." I recall one patient who continued with some incontinence for 18 months before he no longer leaked. It is important that you don't become discouraged after a few weeks. But be aware that there are no guarantees as to whether or not you will leak.

If I leak, does that mean something was done wrong in surgery?

No. It is simply a reflection of how your body healed. I recall some patients who had everything put back together perfectly during surgery but still ended up with some incontinence. Then there have been others who had problems in surgery that left us with expectations of leakage, and they were as dry as a man can be after the catheter came out.

What if I am not leaking?

If you don't leak, consider yourself fortunate. I have had patients who had absolutely no incontinence after the Foley catheter was removed. One patient wasn't worried until he went out to play golf with three other men who also had prostate cancer surgery. In sharing their experiences and problems, he was made to feel that he was supposed to leak, as they did. He felt sure something must be wrong. I had to reassure him during his postoperative checkup that all was well and that he was one of the fortunate ones who had a quick recovery with no leakage.

Are there any medications that can help?

Certain medications and decongestants help to snug up the urethral muscles and may reduce urine leakage. Because these medications possibly can increase your blood pressure, it is a good idea to have your blood pressure checked twice a week. Talk to your doctors about the pros and cons of any recommended medication.

What about the penile clamp?

This is a device that snaps onto the penis and prevents urine leakage. If used at all, it should be used only for short periods of time. If left on the penis too long, damage to the skin and underlying tissues can occur.

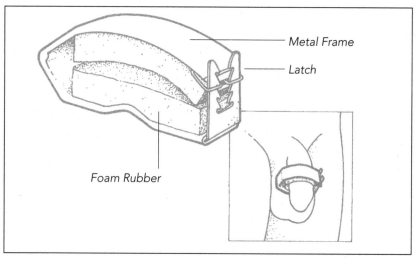

PENILE CLAMP. Penile clamp squeezes the urethra shut to prevent urine from leaking.

I personally don't like to prescribe the penile clamp, and discourage men from using a clamp in the first few months after surgery. I have seen a few patients who have become totally dependent on the clamp. These men stop trying to regain control. They no longer do the Kegel exercises and remain incontinent.

How does it work?
The penile clamp applies direct physical pressure to the urethra, forcing it shut so there is no leakage of urine.

How long can I leave it on?
It is important to take it off about every 30 minutes (to let your bladder empty) and then reapply as needed. This removal will also allow the blood flow to keep tissues healthy. I ask patients to use the clamp only for special occasions, such as going out to dinner, to a movie or to church.

Are there any problems with the clamp?
If you use a clamp too early after surgery and too often, you will not be motivated to work on controlling leakage with Kegel exercises. This excessive reliance can result in permanent problems in controlling your urine.

How soon after surgery can I start using a clamp?
I usually ask that you wait at least six to eight weeks.

What about adult male undergarments?
These are simply large *absorbent underpants*, often with a hole cut out in which the man places his penis. These work by absorbing any urine that leaks. These are usually used in the early phases of recovery after surgery. It is important that you don't become dependent on these and stop trying to control your urine.

Are there any operations to correct incontinence?
Yes. If the leakage is severe and prolonged, the urologist can operate to place a device called an *artificial urinary sphincter (AUS)* or a "male sling." In some cases the procedure for the sling can be done at the time of the prostatectomy.

What is an artificial sphincter?
This is an implanted device that is surgically placed around the urethra, just at the bladder neck. When activated by a pump in the scrotum, this device tightens around the urethra and prevents urine from leaking. This is called "active urethral compression." Most men who receive a sphincter are very happy. The artificial sphincter is best for severe leaking and has a very high degree of patient satisfaction.

How long does the operation take to place the artificial sphincter?
This procedure usually takes just and hour or two, under anesthesia. There can be at least one overnight stay in the hospital.

What is done before a sphincter can be put in?
It is important to have a complete evaluation before surgery to be sure there is normal bladder function and no scarring or other irregularities that may compromise the results. A detailed study of bladder function, called a *urodynamics evaluation*, may be performed. A cystoscopy is usually performed to evaluate the bladder neck visually. We often ask you to keep a "diary" of your day-to-day situation.

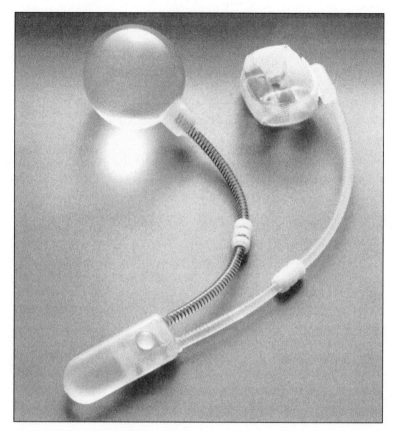

ARTIFICIAL SPHINCTER. Placed surgically, the artificial sphincter provides relief from severe urinary incontinence. The cuff surrounds the bladder neck and urethra and squeezes shut, blocking any urine leakage. The device is activated and deactivated by a pump placed in the scrotum. Photo courtesy of American Medical Systems Inc.

What problems can occur with an artificial sphincter?

Because this is an operation with implantation of a mechanical device, be aware that there are risks for failure or problems. These problems include bleeding, infection around the device, urinary retention, erosion of the device into the urethra, continued incontinence and malfunction or breakage of the artificial sphincter.

These problems occur rarely (in less than 1–3% of patients). Only a small percentage of men may need additional surgery to adjust the device or repair malfunction. It's important for you to be aware of how this device works so you will have realistic expectations.

Because it is a mechanical device, a low percentage of malfunction is expected and unavoidable, and additional surgery can be required.

Are there any factors that increase the risk of problems with the sphincter?
Yes, if you have had prior pelvic radiation, are older than 75, or have significant peripheral vascular disease or diabetes, you are at a higher risk for problems.

What is a "male sling?"
This short outpatient procedure involves placing a strip of material under the internal urethra. This sling is then gently lifted up and secured behind the pubic bone with bone screws or anchors. The sling is best for mild to moderate incontinence (defined as use of about one to two pads a day).

How does lifting the urethra reduce leaking?
This gentle elevation results in enough compression of the urethra in just the right location to eliminate the need for pads in 75% of men and to dramatically reduce leaking in another 20%. This is called "passive urethral compression."

Can any urologist perform the "male sling"?
Currently the best results for most men are with specialists and general urologists who have learned and perfected the technique. As long as your doctor has a good track record with high levels of success you will do well. The long-term results of the male sling appear good.

The sling can be used if there are problems with an artificial urinary sphincter.

Are there any other operations for incontinence?
Yes. Many men are having injections of a bulking agent such as collagen into the bladder neck to try to reduce leakage.

How do collagen injections work?

The collagen is injected through a flexible needle into the tissues at the bladder neck. When successful, this causes the tissues to enlarge (bulk up) and squeeze together to prevent leakage.

What is collagen?

Collagen is the protein extract of connective tissue from cattle. It is injected elsewhere in the body by plastic surgeons as a filler to add shape or fullness.

How many collagen treatments are needed?

Five to seven sessions of collagen injections may be required to achieve control of urine. There is no way to know in advance how many times a person will need treatment.

How long will the collagen last?

If it works, it should be effective for at least a few years. Some men will notice that it gradually becomes less effective over several years. Each individual may have different results. Some may have great urinary control for several months and then notice increased leaking. Others may go many years without problems.

Does collagen injection work for everyone?

No. In fact, as a treatment for urine leakage after a radical prostatectomy, perhaps only a third of patients will notice some improvement. The nice thing is that collagen injections are easy to do as an outpatient procedure, and can be repeated. A real concern is that if the bulking agent does not work, it makes having a sling or artificial sphincter much harder to perform later on with higher risks of problems and complications.

What are the chances I might have an allergic reaction to collagen injections?

This is very rare, but because it can be serious, special precautions are taken, such as a skin test.

TREATMENTS FOR INCONTINENCE

Biofeedback	Penile clamp
Kegel exercises	Collagen injection
Medications	Artificial sphincter
Condom catheter	Male sling

How long should I wait after my prostatectomy to try collagen injections to control urinary leakage?
You should wait at least one year.

Can I have collagen injected if I've also had radiation?
Because of scarring of the tissues, it usually will not work to try to inject collagen if you have had radiation following a radical prostatectomy.

What else can be done if I leak urine?
A device called a *condom catheter* is sometimes used, but I don't recommend it. Placed over the penis, this device catches leaked urine and drains it into a bag. Condom catheters can be associated with many problems, including hard-to-treat urinary-tract infections. Because of this, I strongly discourage the use of condom catheters.

Is biofeedback a treatment option?
Yes, some men who can learn to control their pelvic muscles through biofeedback can have improvement with less urine leakage. Talk to your doctor. There are a number of new advances that teach men how to tighten their pelvic muscles. Though it doesn't work for everyone, I have had several patients with rather dramatic improvement after learning biofeedback.

ERECTILE DYSFUNCTION (IMPOTENCE)—CAUSES AND TREATMENTS

28

W hen considering treatments for prostate cancer, most men have concerns about the potential for impotence and problems with erections as a side effect. With all of the media attention that developed after the release of Viagra, erectile dysfunction (ED) has become a topic of open discussion.

With few exceptions, if you develop prostate cancer, you will have to consider the impact of any and all the treatments on your ability to have an erection. For those men who already have lost the ability to obtain an erection, there is a lot of interest in regaining their potency. Therapy encouraging erections regularly after prostate cancer treatments is called "penile rehab." It is thought that such therapy will allow for quicker return of erections. This chapter will explain some of the treatment options and devices that are available to bring back this part of your sexual life.

What exactly is impotence?
Impotence is the inability to achieve and sustain an adequate erection for sexual intercourse.

What is erectile dysfunction?

Erectile dysfunction is the ability to achieve an erection that may not be as adequate as you might prefer. Your penis might be erect, but the erection may not last long enough before it fades away. *Erectile dysfunction* is a broader term than *impotence*.

How does prostate cancer affect erections?

All aspects of prostate cancer and treatments can impact on erections. Surgery and radiation can damage the nerves and blood vessels that allow men to achieve and maintain an erection. Hormone therapy can often eliminate erections through unknown mechanisms. In addition, a lack of interest in sex can sometimes accompany the loss of testosterone.

The good news is that with all the new and exciting nonsurgical methods of restoring erections, almost everyone can be happy with the final outcome.

Can I become impotent if I choose to do nothing for my prostate cancer?

Yes. Many men describe problems with erections even without any of the curative treatments that are available. It may be that as the cancer grows and spreads, it can grow through the outside of the prostate and damage the nerves that are just outside the gland. Or perhaps it is a result of fears, concerns, anxiety, pain and stress that can go along with prostate cancer. As I tell many of my patients, even ignoring the cancer and trying to forget about it can still lead to erectile problems.

Can I become impotent if I choose radiation?

Yes. Between 25% and 50% of men who undergo radiation therapy will become impotent. Unlike after surgery, where impotence is immediate, radiation may cause problems slowly. Even if they have great erections before, during and after the radiation treatments, many men describe a slow loss of erections over about one year's time. It is believed to be a result of radiation injury to the small blood vessels and nerves. It is hoped that there will be fewer problems with the more focused therapies.

Can I develop erectile problems after interstitial seed therapy?

Yes. Up to 63% of men who have good erections before interstitial seed therapy will have significant problems with erections afterward. Like external-beam therapy, seed therapy can take quite a while to cause loss of erections. The skill of the radiation therapist can impact on your chances for ED.

How does radical surgery actually make a man impotent?

Many times the tiny nerves that transmit messages to get an erection can be cut or damaged when removing the prostate. If the message can't get to the penis to allow blood in, there will be no erections. In addition, there may be injury to the blood supply that helps with erections. Improved techniques for nerve preservation and earlier use of medications such as Viagra are leading to improved results.

Why does hormone therapy eliminate my interest in sex?

The male hormone testosterone is responsible for much of the male sex drive, called *libido*. In addition, testosterone plays an important role in the ability to get an erection. When testosterone is eliminated from the body, it is common for men to become impotent, which is not such a problem because they are no longer interested in sex. This doesn't happen to everyone though. There are some men who are still quite interested in sex and claim they continue to have normal erections.

Why am I still impotent if I had the nerve-sparing radical prostatectomy?

Even if you had the nerves saved, it can still take many months and occasionally up to a year or two for men to gradually regain the ability to have an adequate erection. If only one side of the nerves was saved, then your odds of regaining potency are not great, but it can still happen. This delay may be as a result of injury to the nerves during their preservation. Nerves are very slow to heal.

OPTIONS FOR TREATING IMPOTENCE

Do nothing
Oral medications
Vacuum devices
Penile self-injection

Penile implants
- Bendable (malleable)
- Mechanical
- Inflatable, no separate pump (self-contained)
- Inflatable, separate pump (multicomponent)

How does blocking testosterone make me impotent?

No one really knows. We know that the brain and hormones work together with nerves and blood vessels to bring on an erection. The disruption of that fine balance may be enough to keep an erection from developing.

Can I have an implant at the time of the prostatectomy?

Yes, some doctors simultaneously place a penile implant at the time of the prostatectomy, with excellent results and many happy patients.

Does the quality of my erection before treatment affect whether or not I have erections after treatment?

Definitely, yes. Younger, healthier men with good erections are far more likely to have the return of their erections after surgery or radiation than older men who already had erection problems.

What can I do to regain erections if I am impotent after treatment?

There are several excellent treatment options or devices that you have to choose from to bring back erections like those you used to have when you were younger. These include *Viagra, Levitra, Cialis, vacuum erection devices, penile self-injections* and *penile implants*.

Viagra, Levitra, and Cialis

When first introduced, Viagra (sildenafil) was a revolutionary new medication taken orally to restore erections. Expert Dr. Peter Burrows in Tucson, Arizona, notes that Viagra works by relaxing smooth muscles in the small arteries of the penis, allowing more blood flow and return of erections. Viagra's target is an enzyme found almost exclusively in the penis. Levitra (vardenafil) is similar to Viagra as is Cialis (tadalafil), the longer-acting medication.

Are these oral ED medications safe?

Yes, for most men. As with all medications, there is always the potential for side effects. Though infrequent, these include mild headache, flushing, indigestion and runny nose, and about 3% of men will note a temporary blue haze in their eyesight. It is because of this uncommon change in vision that we ask all pilots (or anyone else whose vision must not be impaired on the job) to not take these medications for a day prior to flying until they see if they have any problems.

Initially, there was a lot of concern about heart patients and these medications. We now know that taking these pills regularly actually reduces a man's risk for heart attacks and death!

Of course, increased exertion with sexual activity can be a problem if you have significant heart disease.

Will these medications improve my interest in sex?

No, they cannot improve your sex drive (libido). They simply serve to improve erections by increasing blood flow.

Does it always work?

No, about a third of men do not have satisfactory improvement with these medications. Be aware that it can take six tries with a specific ED medication before you consider it a failure. Often one medication may not work, while another is very effective. If you still don't get an erection after trying different medications, there may be a serious lack of blood flow or a nerve injury limiting the medication's effectiveness.

Where should I get the specific instructions and precautions about taking Viagra, Levitra or Cialis?

Your doctor and pharmacist should review with you the directions, timing, dosages and precautions associated with any medication. If you have any

?

Are there any medications that I cannot take with Viagra, Levitra or Cialis?

Yes, a category of heart medications called nitrates reacts dangerously with these pills. In fact, most of the problems associated with these medications involved the use of a nitrate at the same time. It turns out that the combination of these nitrates (nitroglycerine, nitrate pastes, long-acting nitrates, isosorbides) with Viagra, Levitra or Cialis can dangerously drop your blood pressure when taken. You must inform your partner, so that if a problem should develop, emergency paramedics and emergency-room doctors will know immediately that you have taken these meds. If they don't know, the emergency personnel might give you nitrates and drop your blood pressure, with potentially fatal consequences. If you take nitrates, then you cannot take Viagra, Levitra or Cialis.

history of an eye disorder called retinitis pigmentosa you should not take any of these medications! Serious eye and vision problems can result.

How soon should I start using Viagra, Levitra or Cialis after my prostatectomy?

Men should begin using these medications a few weeks after surgery to get blood flowing into the penis and start stimulation of the nerves that cause erections. The sooner these nerves begin working, the better the chances for the return of normal erections. The longer you wait, the higher the chances for scarring of the penile tissues. There is truth to the phrase "If you don't use it, you will lose it."

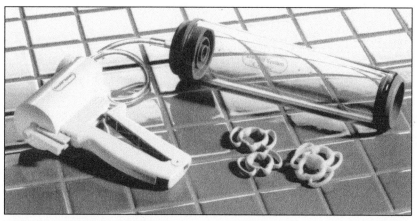

VACUUM ERECTION DEVICE. A vacuum erection device uses a pump attached to a plastic cylinder. The cylinder is placed over the lubricated penis, and a vacuum is created by the pump. This results in blood flowing into the two chambers in the penis that create an erection. An elastic ring is then slipped off of the cylinder onto the base of the penis to keep the blood in place and the erection intact. Photo courtesy of Osbon.

Vacuum Erection Device

How does the vacuum device work?

The first and perhaps easiest option, the *vacuum erection device*, is is a large plastic tube with a pump attached. Placed over your lubricated penis, the pump is activated, creating a vacuum inside the tube. Blood flows into the penis because of the vacuum, giving you a great erection. Then you pull an elastic ring off the tube onto the base of the penis. The ring holds all the blood in the penis, which gives you a good erection until the ring is taken off, up to 30 minutes later.

Why can I leave the ring on for only 30 minutes?

The blood being held inside the penis by the ring is not able to circulate. If the blood is kept in your penis too long, serious problems could develop. Therefore, you need to take the ring off after no more than 30 minutes, but you can always put it back on several minutes later if you need to.

Will the vacuum device work even if the nerves are cut or damaged?

It works in almost everyone, whether or not the nerves are intact or functional. It doesn't rely on the body's ability to pump in blood. It is an external mechanism that achieves the same results.

How often can I use the device?

There are no limits as long as you follow the instructions and take off the ring every 30 minutes.

Does the rubber ring hurt?

It can be tight for some men. There are a number of different-size rings so that over time you'll be able to decide which one works best for you. The ideal ring is one that is not too tight, is not uncomfortable and squeezes enough to maintain an erection to your satisfaction.

Can I still ejaculate with the ring on?

Maybe. If you have had a prostatectomy, there will be no ejaculate as the glands that make the semen have all been removed. If you have had radiation or hormone therapy, then many times you can still ejaculate. Some of the rings are modified to allow for ejaculation.

But don't confuse *orgasm* with *ejaculation*. Ejaculate is the fluid that comes out of the penis during orgasm. Orgasm is a generalized feeling of well-being that occurs at the same time as ejaculation would normally occur. The ring will not prevent orgasm.

What if I have problems or questions regarding the vacuum device?

Some companies offer excellent support services with the product. Some have toll-free telephone numbers to call anytime with questions. Others provide trained representatives who can meet you and work to overcome any problems or concerns. They can also teach you some of the fine points that can't be taught in a video or booklet.

Penile Self-Injections

Self-injection of certain medications into the penis to cause an erection is an effective and safe way to restore erections.

How do self-injections work?

Certain substances allow blood to flow into the penis, resulting in an erection. Researchers developed a technique for a man to inject a tiny amount of these very active substances into one of the two chambers of the penis called the *corpora cavernosa*. Over the next ten to twenty minutes, the valves open up, and both chambers fill with blood, causing the penis to become erect.

What medications are injected?

Urologists use any one or a combination of papaverine, phentolamine or PGE (prostaglandin E). Each doctor has a preferred medication that he or she feels works best with the least problems.

How good are the erections?

When it works, it works great.

How long do the erections last?

Erections from penile injection can last from 30 minutes to two hours.

How often can I do a penile self-injection?

You should limit yourself to about twice a week. Doing this more often increases the risks of scars and penile damage.

How difficult is it to learn how to give myself an injection?

For most men, it is very easy. I teach my patients over three separate visits how to prepare the medication, draw up the syringe to the correct dose and then inject the medication into the corpora safely.

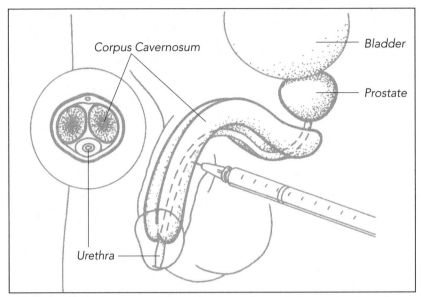

PENILE ANATOMY AND SELF-INJECTION. Normal erection develops when blood flows into both corpora cavernosa within the penis. Penile self-injection is an effective technique to produce an erection by stimulating blood flow with medication injected directly into one of the corpora. After the medication is injected through a tiny needle, blood flow increases and an erection develops.

What can go wrong with a penile injection?
It is possible to develop scarring at the injection site if you use the same place every time. Some men can get a bruise or swelling of the penis if there is bleeding from the injection. The most serious complication is called *priapism*. This is a condition when the erection persists and won't go away. Though this may not sound like a problem, a persistent erection can be very painful and can become a true emergency, requiring immediate treatment.

How often does this happen?
Priapism is quite rare, but it is something you should be aware of.

What should I do if the erection won't fade away?
First, apply an ice pack to your penis. Sometimes this is enough to get the erection to fade away. Never apply the ice directly to your skin. Apply it over a cloth or underwear. If the ice doesn't cause the erection to subside, call your

? *Doesn't the needle hurt?*

No. Most men are surprised when they realize that injecting this medication through a tiny needle into the penis isn't painful at all. Occasionally a patient will complain that his penis ached or was sore, probably from the medication.

urologist *immediately*, even in the middle of the night. Do not wait until the next day! Your doctor may send you to the nearest emergency room for evaluation and treatment.

How long should I wait before calling if the erection persists?

If the erection is still present after several hours, call your urologist immediately. Some doctors want to be called sooner. Others will direct you to call later. You should not wait all night or call after 18 hours to tell your doctor about this problem. The longer you wait, the more difficult it will be to get your erection to go away. It may even require drainage of the blood, with the possible risk of additional problems.

Why is priapism a problem?

If the blood remains in your penis too long, it begins to lose oxygen and starts to thicken. The blood may turn into a dark sludge if you wait too long. This blood is harder to circulate and may damage the delicate tissues inside the penis, making future erections a concern.

Other Injections

What about testosterone injections?

No. Even if your testosterone is low, testosterone injections or patches are not effective for ED after prostate cancer treatments. There is always some worry that if a small speck of tumor is remaining, then testosterone may stimulate the cancer's growth. However, newer studies by Dr. Abraham Morgentaler suggest that, in fact, some men may actually benefit from testosterone therapy without any risk for prostate cancer spread.

Penile Implants

Surgically placed *penile implants*, also called *prostheses*, offer an excellent alternative to the more conservative options discussed for overcoming erectile dysfunction.

These permanent implants are inserted into the chambers of the penis (corpora cavernosa) under a brief anesthesia. As with any mechanical device, there is always the inherent risk of malfunction or breakage of the implant. According to the world's expert in penile implants, Dr. Steven Wilson, penile implants are some of the most dependable medical devices implanted into the human body. The current statistics are that three-year freedom from breakage is 98% and fifteen-year freedom is 70%. This is better freedom from reoperation than surgery for hips, knees, pacemakers, breasts, shoulder implants or implants of virtually any other device.

With penile implants, regardless of type, there is usually a small loss of length from the size of a natural erection. Nevertheless, girth is the most important determinant for penile rigidity, and girth is enhanced from a natural erection. Perhaps best of all is that the individual can keep the erection for as long as he and his partner wish. As with any surgery, finding the most experienced surgeon will give you the best chances for good results with the least risks and complications.

There are two main categories of implants. You can choose between a *bendable* or an *inflatable* implant. The bendable has stiffness but no change in girth and is somewhat difficult to conceal. The inflatable is the most natural, being undetectable in both flaccidity and erection.

Bendable (Malleable) Implant. The bendable or "malleable" prosthesis is usually a collection of silver wires braided inside a silicone sheath or a unique apparatus like a string of pearls on a wire covered with a silicone sheath. It is the simplest type of implant and the least likely to break. The problem with it is that the penis is permanently rigid. It can be bent to aid with urination and concealment. This is the least expensive product and quickest to put in. Because most patients have insurance or Medicare to cover the cost of implantation, they are better served with an inflatable device that has better satisfaction and excellent reliability.

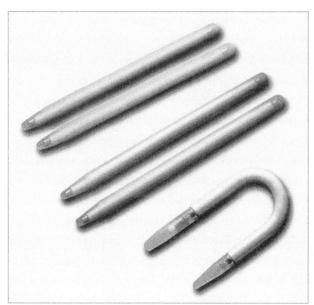

MALLEABLE PENILE IMPLANT. A bendable prosthesis placed into both of the corpora can be bent in any direction. There are no moving parts, so problems with malfunction and breakage are rare. Photos courtesy American Medical Systems Inc.

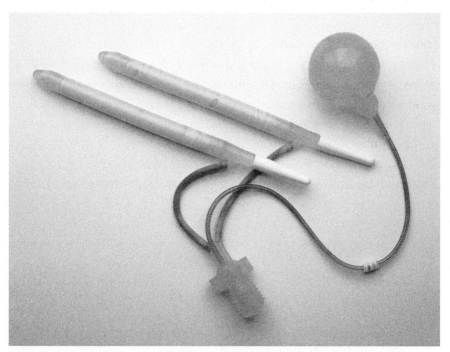

MULTICOMPONENT INFLATABLE PENILE IMPLANT. The inflatable penile implant uses a separate pump placed in the scrotum to inflate and deflate separate cylinders in the corpora. A separate reservoir is implanted to hold fluid. This device allows for the most natural results and is remarkably free of the necessity for repair. Photos courtesy American Medical Systems Inc.

Inflatable (Multicomponent with Pump). This type of device provides an erection that is the most like a natural erection and is totally invisible in the body. Dr. Wilson notes that 80% of the implants done in the United States are the inflatable. It uses a separate pump placed in the scrotum between the testicles with a large reservoir to hold saltwater to provide the erection. The pump is repeatedly squeezed, which transfers fluid from the reservoir into two cylinders. This implant significantly increases penis diameter, sometimes making it even wider than the patient experienced with a natural erection. Lengthening cylinders that will elongate the penis upon inflation are also available. Unfortunately, the lengthening cylinders can prevent shortening seen with semi-rigid rods but will never exceed the length of a natural erection. The penis is relaxed by squeezing a release valve, evacuating the fluid from the cylinders, achieving a very natural flaccidity. While mechanical failures occur rarely, the devices are some of the most dependable products implanted into humans. Infection was formerly a complication, but the addition of antibiotics to the devices has virtually eliminated this problem.

How are the devices inserted?
These products can be put inside the corpora cavernosa through a small incision between the penis and scrotum. The inside of each chamber in the penis is stretched open to allow placement of the device. The chambers are then closed and the skin stitched closed.

How long will I be in the hospital to have an implant?
These are usually done as outpatient procedures or perhaps with a brief overnight stay.

PENILE IMPLANT COMPARISON

Malleable
- Bendable
- Slight increase in penis diameter
- Always rigid (can be bent)

Inflatable (multicomponent)
- Most like normal
- Increase/decrease rigidity
- Slight increase in length and diameter

Is there a lot of pain after surgery?

A patient will often be sore for a while, but it shouldn't be too painful. The pain will gradually subside over time and should easily be handled with oral pain medications.

How soon can I use the implant after surgery?
According to Dr. Wilson, it is best if you wait about four to six weeks to allow the incision to heal before having sexual intercourse. There is some variability depending on which implant model and style you have chosen.

How often can the device break or malfunction?
Though uncommon, any of the devices can break or fail. This is an unavoidable possibility with any mechanical device.

Are there any devices that will not malfunction?
No. Even the most basic malleable device with no moving parts can still develop cracks in the silver wires. No mechanical device is 100% free of risk from malfunction.

What are other possible complications that can occur with penile implants?
Erosion. Erosion is the protrusion of the implant through the end of the penis or urethra. This can occur if your body rejects the device, if it is put in incorrectly or if there is a weakness or breakdown of the surrounding tissue or urethra. Erosion is distinctly more common with semi-rigid devices because of the constant pressure of the semi-rigid device.

Infection. Formerly a big problem, this complication has been virtually eliminated by coating the implant components with antibiotics.

Pain. Patients may complain of pain as a result of the device putting pressure on surrounding tissues, but this is rare.

COSTS OF TREATING IMPOTENCE

OPTION	COST
Nothing	$0
Vacuum device	$300–$500
Penile self-injection	Medication: $40 per Caverject
	Initial office visit: $300–$500
Implants	Bendable: $5,000–$11,000
	Inflatable: $15,000–$25,000

Unsatisfactory results. The results are never as good as you might remember from your own natural erections. Some men are unhappy with the device because of unrealistic expectations. Although most men are happy, there are others who, for a variety of reasons, regret having the device implanted. The implant can be removed without undue harm to the penile tissues. The patient can use a vacuum device after implant removal.

How much do these devices cost?

Including surgical and anesthesia fees, hospitalization and the device itself, charges can range from $5,000 to $25,000 or more. The more elaborate the implant, the more expensive it is. Charges are usually much higher in big cities and on either coast.

What does Medicare cover?

All penile implants are covered. If you have Medicare and a supplement, generally there is no out-of-pocket expense.

What options are covered by private insurance or HMOs?

No preoperative authorization is needed for Medicare, although many other third-party payers require that the physician write for permission.

*Should I be concerned about a silicone reaction or other problems
from the implant material?*

No. In the many hundreds of thousands of men who have had implants placed, there has never been a scientifically documented reaction to the solid silicone material used to make the implants.

Everyone realizes that these implants are placed in an aging population where naturally occurring health problems and diseases increase in frequency. The implant devices do not cause the health problems. Rather, the problems are just coincidental to the implants because both are present in older men.

What if I leak urine and am impotent?

Some men opt for dual implants—both a penile prosthesis and an artificial urinary sphincter—with great success for many of them.

WHAT IS THE RIGHT TREATMENT FOR ME?

29

Every patient and doctor would love to know the right treatment for a man with prostate cancer. Unfortunately, this isn't possible. All we can do is use our experience, our knowledge, the literature and a little common sense to make an educated guess about what would be best for each patient. Too often we struggle, trying to determine which treatment alone will provide the best results for the long term.

Honestly, though, all we can do is help the patient to make the best treatment choice for himself and then be there to advise and counsel should questions or concerns arise along the way.

Deciding on the type of treatment is the bottom-line question for each patient. If we could know what each patient's future holds, and what is really going on in his prostate, then the answers would be easy. But no one knows what tomorrow holds for any of us.

I had a 62-year-old patient who had a flawless prostatectomy with excellent final pathology results. For all intents and purposes, he should have lived a long time.

But two years later, without warning, he had a massive heart attack and died. He had no personal or family history of heart disease. Yet this was "his time to go." Had we known the heart attack was going to happen, we probably would have told him not to do anything for the cancer.

On the other extreme, I had a very ill 79-year-old patient who was diagnosed with prostate cancer. Because of his poor health and limited anticipated life span, the patient, his primary-care doctor and I all agreed we would simply follow him without treatment. After all, we didn't want to do any harm.

Well, this gentleman surprised everyone and lived for several years, long enough to have continued growth and progression of his cancer until it became significant. He hasn't yet died of the cancer, but he may very well have problems from it because we were so conservative.

How can I know what treatment is right or wrong for me?

I find it interesting that with prostate cancer, everyone expects that we will have all the answers and know for an individual what the "right" course of treatment will be. Yet with every other aspect of health, men and women are accustomed to not knowing these answers.

Questions like "Should I choose a heart-bypass operation or not?" or "Should I have my hernia fixed before it becomes an emergency?" or "Should I have my abdominal aneurysm corrected before it can burst and kill me?" are common. Patients and physicians generally understand that it is essentially impossible to give "right" or "wrong" answers to these questions, because the answers must be qualified by the *possible benefits* and *potential risks*.

But with prostate cancer, there is a general expectation that unless we have proof beyond a reasonable doubt that treatments will give you better results, many men should consider just ignoring that they have a potentially lethal disease.

There is no right or wrong. Rather, the question should be "What is best for me at this time?"

How long can I take to choose a treatment?

There really isn't a time limit. You should take the time to gather the information you need to make an intelligent decision. Try to avoid rushing into a snap decision. Most of my patients decide within a few weeks what treat-

What if I change my mind about treatment?

It depends on what you've chosen to do for your prostate cancer. If you've chosen to do nothing and there is evidence that the cancer has spread, then you may still be able to opt for the choices previously presented to you.

If you've chosen surgery as a treatment, you have the option of changing your mind right up until the day of surgery. If you are having second thoughts, then you should talk with your doctor right away.

When you have started radiation, you should finish all the treatments.

If you are having hormone shots, you could choose to change over and have the surgical removal of the testicles. It is not safe or wise to stop the hormone therapy unless told to do so by your doctor.

ment they wish to pursue. Plan to take time to seek out informed and expert opinions.

I have had patients who chose to postpone treatment until after a wedding, a cruise that was already planned, a military reunion and things of that nature. If it is a delay of a few months, then it probably won't make any difference as far as whether or not the cancer will progress during that time. Of course, there's no way to know for certain and there are no guarantees.

If you are going to postpone treatment for several months or more, as a few of my patients have done, then you may want to consider going on the hormone shots once a month just to keep the cancer in check. If you have an aggressive, high-risk cancer, some doctors would encourage pretreatment with hormone shots to make the radiation more effective and control the cancer while awaiting therapy.

The point to remember is that there are *no guarantees* the cancer won't spread during a significant delay of treatment.

Is there any way to know when the cancer will spread so I can hold off treatment until that time?

It would be nice if we could tell if and when the cancer was going to spread. At the present time, this is not possible with any certainty. We know that most of the time, the higher the PSA levels, the more aggressive the cancer. We also know that the more volume of cancer seen, the more likely the cancer is going to or has already started to grow through the capsule or spread to distant sites.

COSTS OF TREATMENTS

30

The majority of men with prostate cancer are fortunate to be insured through Medicare or a health plan. Some have large deductibles, while others have limited or no insurance. It would be ideal if cost were not important in your decision-making, but in reality it can be.

Often, the fear of unknown costs and an incomplete understanding of your own insurance coverage can interfere with your judgment. A few men gamble with time and find themselves very ill, with no insurance, and not yet eligible for Medicare.

Are treatment costs standardized, or do they vary a lot?
Actual costs vary quite a bit from one location to another. Costs tend to be a lot higher in big cities and on the coasts. Perhaps more importantly, the doctors' and hospitals' own costs to provide the medical services tend to be quite a bit more with higher overhead and expenses.

Ask your urologist about the expected costs in your community for the services you are considering. You should also talk with the hospital and with radiation therapists regarding their charges before the treatment starts.

In general, new radiation techniques including IMRT and seeds will cost about the same as or less than surgery, because these techniques avoid hospitalization. The ball-park cost for IMRT can be about $20,000 to $50,000.

Radioactive seed-implant therapy can cost from $15,000 up to $25,000. Radical prostatectomy, with hospital and doctors' fees (including the anesthesiologist, pathologist and assistant surgeon) will run $15,000 to $35,000 or more. Lap robotic surgery may cost a little more because of the use of the robot and more disposable equipment, but with shorter hospitalization. I have heard of fees as high as $140,000 for proton beam with combined external radiation therapies. Therefore, you need to ask your insurance about your particular plan's coverage of various services and treatments.

How much of the cost will I be responsible for?

If you belong to an HMO, you may owe nothing, as long as the treatment is done by the HMO-designated doctor at a contracted facility. The entire workup and procedure will require HMO approval before it can be done.

Medicare will pay 80% of its approved amount for eligible patients. This is what they declare to be reasonable and customary, even though it may be neither. If you have a supplemental or secondary insurance, it will usually pick up the majority of the 20% balance owed, after you have paid your deductible. Medicare tends to pay about 60% of the actual community standard payment.

Whatever the cost, you should choose the treatment that is best for you. It is always sad when patients make a decision based on their finances and expenses. Talk openly to your doctor about possible financial concerns or problems. We may be able to work as your advocate to get you a special rate at the hospital or with other doctors, but if we don't know there is a financial problem, we can't help you.

SECOND OPINION— A GOOD IDEA

31

I t is always a good idea to get a second medical opinion before you make a final decision if you have questions or concerns about your prostate disease and your treatment options. With prostate cancer, you have time to think about treatments and to seek additional opinions. Many insurance companies *require* a second opinion, although this is often waived for cancer treatment and surgery.

This book provides some basic information and background to assist you in making a decision, but it cannot and should not be used to take the place of a qualified physician who can individualize your specific situation and develop recommendations based on the facts.

Will I insult or upset my doctor if I ask for a second opinion?

Be aware that some doctors may feel insulted or hurt if, after spending an hour going over all the details and options with you, you say you want a second opinion. It is important to tell your doctor that you appreciate the time and effort given and that you respect and trust his or her opinion. But make it clear that before you finalize your decision, you would like to speak with another urologist and/or radiation therapist. Most doctors will encourage you to talk to as many other specialists as you need to feel good about making a decision. In my practice, I also encourage my patients to talk with their primary-care physician as well.

What if my urologist doesn't want me to get a second opinion?

You have a right to understand why your doctor is trying to limit your access to another opinion. He may think that what he's telling you is true, and so there's no reason to get another opinion. He may be concerned that another clinic or institution may try to do the surgery and not send you back to him. He may also be concerned that you may end up being swayed by irrelevant information or see a doctor who really isn't experienced dealing with your disease. Whatever the reason, talk with your doctor and reassure him that you intend to return if you choose surgery.

How do I find names of other urologists or doctors for second opinions?

You should not see another urologist in the same group of doctors. If the second doctor disagrees with the recommendations of his partner, he may be reluctant to tell you. Talk with other urologists who do a large number of radical prostatectomies and who are well respected. Be aware that not all urologists do many of these operations, and some don't do them at all. Some will do several operations each week, while others may do only a few each year. Often, your urologist will be able to provide names of other urologists in the community who he respects. You can also ask your primary-care doctor, the local medical society or the local chapter of the American Cancer Society.

What kind of doctor should I talk to for a second opinion?

Ideally, you should talk with physicians who are experienced with prostate cancer and have a good working relationship with specialists from all fields. I prefer to send my patients to another urologist if radical surgery is an option. If you are considering radiation therapy, then definitely you need to talk with a *radiation therapist*. If the cancer is advanced, you may want to meet with a *medical oncologist*, a specialist who treats many cancers with medications, chemotherapy and hormones.

If every doctor advises you to have surgery, then you should strongly consider surgery. If they can't agree, then go back to your urologist and ask why. Perhaps it will be necessary for the specialists and your primary-care doctor to get together to discuss your case so they can come to an agreement about what is best for you.

Each doctor will look at your situation from his or her own personal and professional biases. Take everything with a grain of salt. If every doctor advises you to have surgery, then you should strongly consider surgery. If they can't agree, then go back to your urologist and ask why. Perhaps it will be necessary for the specialists and your primary-care doctor to get together to discuss your case so they can come to an agreement about what is best for you.

Should I talk with my primary-care doctor for his or her recommendations?

Yes, this is always important. He or she should be able to tell you whether or not you are a good candidate for surgery and whether your expected life span is long enough to make surgery worthwhile. I always try to refer patients back to their primary-care doctor for a general medical evaluation and medical clearance before surgery. If my patients don't have a primary-care doctor, then I will provide names of several doctors with whom I work and whose opinions and clinical judgment I respect.

Don't most insurance companies require second opinions for surgery?

Many private insurance plans require a second opinion for *elective noncancer procedures*. Surgery for cancer usually does not need a second opinion. If you are uncertain, call your insurance company and ask. Record the name of the person you speak to and the date and time that you called. Occasionally, insurance companies change their requirements.

What should I do to prepare for a second opinion?
To get the most from a second opinion, take with you all the necessary records so the doctor can know what has happened to you. These records should include (1) the pathology report, (2) PSA test results (old ones as well as the most recent), (3) copies of reports on the bone scan and/or CT scan, if performed, (4) your past medical history and (5) a list of medications you are currently taking.

If you ask your original doctor to forward your records to the doctor providing the second opinion, call the office of the second-opinion doctor a few days before your appointment to confirm that the records have indeed arrived. The best way to ensure that your records are there is to bring them with you. Give your original doctor plenty of time to copy the records for you.

Should I bring just the reports or do I need the X-rays?
Bring the actual X-ray films with the reports, not just the reports. You should also bring the actual glass pathology slides, which you can get from the pathology office that reads the slides. Although it usually isn't necessary, some urologists (especially at teaching institutions) prefer to have their own pathologists and residents look at the slides. They will usually return the slides and films for you, after your appointment.

How do I obtain the X-ray films and pathology slides?
Well in advance, you will need to go to the facilities where the X-rays or scans were taken and sign a release. Sometimes the films will be at your original doctor's office, but he or she won't be able to give them to you. The general rule is that your doctor will have to return the films to the X-ray facility, which can then check them out to you. You should also contact the pathology lab to pick up the slides or to have them sent to you, if the lab is located out of town.

Will the doctor providing the second opinion write to my original doctors?
If you want your second-opinion report sent to your doctors, give the doctor the names and addresses of those doctors so that a full report of the second opinion can be sent to them.

Should I travel to a well-known institution for my surgery or radiation?

Probably not. If you are in a relatively rural area, or if you have a limited choice of urologists, then you may want to travel to a big-name facility. Otherwise, it is unlikely that the care in a far-off medical center is really any better than what's available in your own community. I spent two years of my training at a well-known medical center with an international reputation. We often wondered why some patients would travel long distances to see us, when some of the best doctors were in their own hometowns.

In other words, you shouldn't have to travel to get good care. Many of the country's leading urology residents often move to smaller communities or even rural areas to avoid the politics or fast pace of the big cities. Whether or not you need to go elsewhere should be dictated by whether the quality of care you need is available at home. You will often be wrong if you assume the level of care elsewhere is better.

What if my children want me to have my surgery where they live?

This happens a lot. Children decide the urologist in their community is better than the one you are seeing. Obviously, they can't really know anything about your doctor, but still they may try to pressure you to travel to their hometown for your surgery or radiation. They may explain they need to be around during your recovery. Many people feel loyal to their own doctor and thus will try to persuade you to see their surgeon.

My advice is for you to make your own decision about who will be your physician. Your recovery shouldn't require any special care or assistance. In other words, you decide where you will have your treatment and thank your children for their concern.

Can I bring my wife or other family members with me to my second-opinion appointment?

Absolutely—yes. I strongly encourage my patients to bring anyone whose opinion will be important in making a decision about treatment options. In fact, I am somewhat disappointed when the patient shows up alone for his consultation. I once had such a large family show up to participate that we had to use the office lobby to handle everyone.

What if the doctor can't see me for a second opinion for several weeks or more?
This is usually the case. A few weeks won't hurt anything. It is better to get a regular appointment than to try to squeeze in a "quickie" opinion that may be inadequate to discuss your situation. Rarely is there a biologic urgency to be treated. Take the time to do whatever you need to feel confident about the treatment you have selected.

> *It is extremely important that you choose a physician you trust and feel good about.*

What if the doctor providing the second opinion wants to do the surgery?
Although there are no laws regarding this, it is considered by many to be *unethical* for the doctor providing the second opinion to try to "steal" you as a patient. Sometimes, they can be subtle by suggesting they can do a better job. Sometimes they don't even ask—they just tell you that you have been scheduled for surgery or radiation. Be wary of this.

Some referral centers depend on doing the surgery following second opinions. Watch out for the "factory approach." Before you realize it, the treatment is finished and you're leaving the hospital. Unfortunately, this happens all too often. If you believe the services in your area are not good enough, talk to your doctors honestly for a referral to a regional center or to a urologist in a larger community.

If you truly feel more confident with the physician providing the second opinion, then you should tell both the original doctor and the second doctor how you feel. Explain why you have decided to change doctors. Some doctors will not take over your care unless the first doctor resigns as your treating physician, even if you *want* the second doctor to assume your care.

If I'm giving a second opinion, I always try to send the patient back to his urologist unless the patient has very personal and legitimate reasons for wanting me to assume his care. It is extremely important that you choose a physician you trust and feel good about.

HOW TO FIND A GOOD UROLOGIST

32

Then here isn't an easy way to find the "best" urologist. You obviously want to have the best urologist available taking care of you if you have prostate cancer, but you will usually have to depend on your primary-care doctor for a referral.

Sometimes the best urologist may not be the most personable. Also, the best doctors will not be the easiest to see on short notice. Take the time to make an appointment to see the doctor when he can spend the necessary time with you. Occasionally patients will "sneak" in more quickly than they should by claiming to have some urgent problem that needs attention immediately. Don't use this as an excuse to get an appointment.

The potential problem in my office is that I set aside about 60 to 90 minutes to talk with someone about prostate cancer and the treatment options available. If another patient squeezes in because he wants urgent attention, there is no way I can give the first patient all the time and attention he needs. Such schedule interruptions can ruin the day for the next 15 patients who did wait weeks for their appointment that day.

Don't be alarmed or surprised if you have to wait. Actually, it is a good sign if the doctor has a waiting list of several weeks or more. In my practice, nonurgent patients can sometimes wait several weeks for an appointment. If you have a truly urgent problem or if your primary-care doctor calls over to get you in sooner, then my office has a policy of trying to find a time slot somewhere.

Be patient with your doctor. It may be worth the extra wait to see a doctor who will be honest and straightforward and won't try to push you in a direction that isn't right.

Who will my primary-care doctor refer me to for urology treatment?

Your primary-care doctor will usually give you the names of several urologists to whom he refers his patients. But be aware that a doctor on this list may or may not be the best one for you.

In the real world, doctors get set in their referral patterns and usually don't refer to another specialist even if the other doctor may be better. In fact, the quality of the care provided is not usually a factor in the referral. Often doctors will refer to others of a similar age group. Young doctors tend to refer to other young doctors, while older doctors tend to keep referring to the other doctors of similar age and training.

Your HMO or insurance plan may have contracted urology specialists for referral. If the urologist in the HMO isn't the best or if you don't get along, you are essentially stuck unless there are several to choose from.

Does it matter if my urologist is younger or older?

Some patients like doctors recently out of training, thinking they will be up-to-date on new techniques and treatments. Other patients prefer older physicians with experience and wisdom.

The truth is that it is the quality of the individual physician that counts. Age is irrelevant. There are some young physicians with experience, wisdom and common sense, while there may be older physicians who are very current on the newest procedures and techniques. Don't prejudge a urologist solely on age.

So how do I find the best urologist in my area?

To find the best urologist in your community, talk to your friends and ask for names. This is how I ultimately developed the list of specialists to whom

I refer my friends and family. I just ask many fellow doctors who they like, and slowly a few names rise to the top.

Find out who is liked, and just as important, who isn't liked. Ask why. Does the doctor explain everything, or does he or she just tell you that you need an operation and turn you over to a nurse to set it up?

Talk to nurses, especially those who work in the operating rooms, in the recovery rooms or on the surgical floors. Call your county medical society. Call the local chapter of the American Cancer Society.

When you have a name, you can contact your state board of medical examiners to see if there have been a large number of lawsuits against the urologist. Most urologists will have had a few lawsuits in their careers, which does not necessarily suggest wrongdoing. Instead, the lawsuits often indicate bitter patients who are unhappy with outcomes of treatment that the urologist had no control over.

Are there specific qualities that I should look for in a doctor?

Be concerned about any doctor who won't answer your questions or seems bothered or annoyed that you are interested in a conversation rather than a lecture. This could mean the doctor is insecure with his or her own knowledge or skills. It may also mean the doctor is insulted that you don't trust him or her to make all your decisions.

I have many patients who left their original doctor because the doctor refused to answer questions or became upset when they demonstrated they had done some reading on the subject of prostate cancer.

Watch out for any doctor who tries to corner you into making a snap decision about your care or insists that he or she is the only one capable of caring for you.

What if my doctor is not listed as a board-certified specialist?

When you check on the credentials of a doctor, make sure you are using an up-to-date information resource.

I recently had a patient who was concerned that I was not board-certified. He had checked into my credentials through a friend who had a book of surgical specialists. As I sat and looked at my Certificate of Board Certification, I confirmed to myself that I was indeed board-certified and then asked my

What does being "board-certified" mean?

This is a *voluntary* examination to maintain and promote a basic level of knowledge in the specialty. In urology in the United States, this examination is monitored by the American Board of Urology. In Canada, it is the Royal College of Physicians and Surgeons, located in Ontario. Each country has its own certification process.

patient how old the reference book was. Obviously, it was several years older than my certification.

What does a doctor have to do to be board-certified?

The certification process is a very intense experience in which the urologist first must provide a detailed log of every surgery performed for at least 12 months. If this list is deemed adequate, then the doctor is required to take a two-day written and oral exam. If the doctor passes all parts of the exams, he or she will be certified by the board. Many doctors are required to take a renewal exam each decade to maintain their certification.

How can I find out if my doctor is board-certified?

In the United States, the American Board of Urology awards a certificate to urologists who become board-certified. This certificate will be displayed in your doctor's office. You can call 1-866-275-2267 or go to www.abms.com to check a doctor's board certification. In Canada, board certification is provided by the Royal College of Physicians and Surgeons of Canada, 1-613-730-8177.

If the doctor is board-certified, does that mean he or she is a good urologist?

It means the doctor has a good fund of knowledge and was able to pass written and oral exams about different aspects of urology and urologic surgery. However, good judgment and operating skill are two things that cannot be measured by this certification process.

I know of excellent doctors who had problems, not with their skills and knowledge, but with the examination process. In general, board certification does assure the community that the urologist at least has a good fund of knowledge. There's more to being a good doctor than being board-certified.

Are doctors board-certified for life?

This depends on the specialty and when they took the exam. Urologists who became board-certified *before* the mid-1980s are board-certified forever. They are not required to retake the certification test ever again. Urologists who were first board-certified in the mid-1980s or later are required to retake the exam every ten years to maintain board-certification status.

Should I go to a urologist at a university hospital?

You shouldn't select a physician just because he or she is affiliated with a university teaching or research setting. You may have heard that you should get your care only in a university system. It's been said that university doctors are well-published, authors of many articles and books and therefore must know more about surgery.

As far as the publishing of articles and books is concerned, there is no correlation between surgical skill and how well a doctor speaks or how many articles and books he may have written. The doctor should be judged on his or her own merits. Whether he or she practices in a community setting or at a powerful university teaching center has nothing to do with the doctor's skills.

What you really want is a caring and compassionate urologist, technically excellent, with a good track record, outstanding judgment, a history of minimal complications and happy patients and referring doctors.

inventory management system.

Opened music CDs/DVDs/audio books may not be returned, and can be exchanged only for the same title and only if defective. NOOKs purchased from other retailers or sellers are returnable only to the retailer or seller from which they are purchased, pursuant to such retailer's or seller's return policy. Magazines, newspapers, eBooks, digital downloads, and used books are not returnable or exchangeable. Defective NOOKs may be exchanged at the store in accordance with the applicable warranty.

Returns or exchanges will not be permitted (i) after 14 days or without receipt or (ii) for product not carried by Barnes & Noble or Barnes & Noble.com.

Policy on receipt may appear in two sections.

YOU MAY ALSO LIKE...

Prostate Cancer For Dummies
by Paul H. Lange

Dr. Patrick Walsh's Guide to Surviving...
by Patrick C. Walsh

How We Survived Prostate Cancer: What We...
by Victoria Hallerman

The Cleveland Clinic Guide to Prostate...
by Eric Klein

The Prostate Cancer Treatment Book
by Peter Grimm

QUESTIONS TO ASK YOUR DOCTOR

33

I t is a good idea to ask a lot of questions and keep a record of your progress when you are being treated for prostate cancer. You should also write down the answers you get. Better yet, ask your doctor to write down the answers next to the questions. Some doctors even advocate recording the consultation so you can go back and review the discussion later on. Here are some key questions to ask your urologist or primary-care doctor.

1. What is my PSA level?
   a. Does it fall within the "normal" range for my age?
   b. What were the levels of my past PSA tests?
2. Has my PSA level changed significantly over time (PSA velocity)?
3. Is there a reason to recheck the PSA in eight to twelve weeks? (A recent infection or catheter might be a reason.)
4. What is the grade and volume of cancer in the biopsies and how significant are they? What do you think about getting a second pathology opinion on the biopsy specimens? What is the likelihood for under- or over-grading?
5. What did the bone scan show? (If one was done.)
6. What were the results of the CT scan or MRI? (If one was done.)

7. What is the clinical stage of cancer and how significant is that?

8. Do you think the cancer is curable with a single therapy or multiple therapies?

   a. What are the chances that the cancer has spread to the lymph nodes?

9. What are the treatment options available for me?

10. What are the chances the cancer will progress if it is left untreated? Over what time?

11. If radical prostatectomy is an option, who will do it? (If your doctor is a urologist, he or she probably will do it.) What technique do you recommend? Why? Will you remove my lymph nodes?

12. How many of these operations do you do in a year? (Twenty-five or more is good.)

13. Are resident physicians involved in the surgery or postoperative care?

    a. If yes, what exactly do they do in the surgery?

    b. What year of training after medical school are they in? (In other words, how many years of postgraduate training have they had?)

    c. What specialty training are these residents in? (Sometimes residents may rotate their training among various specialties.)

14. Do you use autologous blood transfusions during prostate surgery? (Because autologous blood—donated by the patient for his own use is so infrequently needed for transfusions, some doctors don't even ask for this.)

15. How often do you give blood transfusions during surgery? (Should be used very rarely.)

16. After surgery, do your patients go to the intensive care unit (ICU)? (Ideally, this should be almost never.)

17. How many days do your patients usually stay in the hospital, not counting the surgical day? (This should be from one to three days, depending on the procedure.)

18. What percentage of your patients have severe, permanent incontinence after treatment? (This should be around 1% to 3%.)

19. Are you board-certified? When did you take the exam? (Remember, some older urologists were "grandfathered" in so they automatically have certification for life. More recently trained urologists have to take recertification tests every ten years).

20. Do you use an epidural anesthetic during surgery? For how long? Do you use a PCA pump?

21. How long do you leave the Foley catheter in after surgery?

22. How often should I expect to see you for follow-up visits after I go home?

23. Who will do the long-term follow-up after my treatment? (This is an important question, especially if you belong to an HMO where the primary-care doctor may actually follow your treatment, hopefully at the direction of the urologist.)

24. How soon can I go back to work or resume normal activities, such as golf, tennis, gardening or bike riding? (The answers will vary depending on your procedure.)

25. Will I be admitted to the hospital the day before or the day of surgery? (Most admit the morning of surgery.)

26. What kind of preparation for surgery will I need? (This might include bowel-prep enemas or antibiotics.)

27. How soon should I have the surgery after learning I have cancer? (It is never an emergency. Be wary if a doctor tries to push you through quickly, before you have a chance to think about treatment options.)

28. If radiation is recommended, how soon should I start the radiation? How long can I wait to start? Do you want me to continue or stop taking antioxidants during radiation?

29. After surgery or radiation, how long should I wait to see if I can still get a normal erection before I seek treatment for impotence? Can I start taking the ED meds right away?

30. After radiation or surgery, how long should I wait to consider treatment options for urinary incontinence?

31. Do you believe in early or late treatment of advanced prostate cancer? (I prefer early. Some doctors like to wait until the cancer is causing problems.)

32. Which type of hormone treatment do you prefer and why? Will you check my testosterone levels to be sure the hormone therapy is working?

33. Do you believe in the use of antiandrogens? When do you start these?

FOLLOW-UP AFTER TREATMENT

34

F ollow-up care will be necessary for the rest of your life after you've been treated for prostate cancer. If the cancer does return, early detection and treatment can make a difference.

Today, the PSA blood test is the best and least expensive way of making sure that the cancer hasn't come back after treatment. As long as the PSA level remains stable, you are doing fine. How often you need to be seen depends on your particular medical situation, the final grade and stage of the cancer, the treatment you received and how likely it is that the cancer was cured.

Initially after radiation or surgery, you will probably need to get the PSA rechecked every three to four months for the first year, then every four to six months the next year or two, then every six to twelve months thereafter. The longer you go after treatment without signs of cancer recurrence, the longer you can go between PSA checks.

What happens if the PSA goes up?
The answer will depend on how much change there has been in the PSA, to what level and over how much time. You should remember there is some fluctuation in lab testing.

Minor changes probably don't mean anything. But if the PSA continues to rise with each recheck, then it means the cancer has come back. The faster the climb, the more concerned we are. You may even need additional treatments. A PSA doubling time (how fast the PSA doubles) is another

> *If the cancer does return, early detection and treatment can make a difference.*

key measure of the aggressiveness of the cancer. The faster the cancer is growing, the shorter the doubling time. A rapid increase suggests that the cancer not only is back but is growing vigorously. Sometimes the PSA elevation is so small and so slow, we choose to just watch it over time.

Should I worry if the PSA level starts to go up after surgery?

Not initially. Before I become worried, I would want to get a repeat test result. If the PSA continues to rise, it usually means that there is some recurrent prostate cancer. No one really knows when and if additional treatments should be started. In my practice, if the PSA goes up rapidly, then I'm more inclined to recommend either "salvage" radiation treatment to the pelvis or hormone therapy. At a PSA of 1 or 2, I usually recommend treatment.

What should the PSA be after a radical prostatectomy?

The PSA level should be 0.0. We hope there is no more cancer or prostate tissue left behind. No other tissues can produce a significant amount of PSA. Sometimes the PSA is reported as less than 0.3 or 0.5. These basically mean the same thing. It's just the lab's way of reporting the result. Some lab machines don't try to determine the exact amount if it is at a very low, almost undetectable level. Occasionally the report will come back at 0.1 or 0.2. Lab tests are not perfect. There are some minor variations in lab testing that are always present and unavoidable. After surgery, many specialists prefer to order a supersensitive PSA.

It's not good that the surgery wasn't curative. If your prostate contained high-grade disease (Gleason sum 8, 9 or 10) then you are at a higher risk of recurrence, and should consider additional treatments.

What should the PSA level be after radiation?

Unlike surgery where the PSA should be 0.0, after radiation the PSA usually slowly drops down to a level ideally *below* 0.5. The longer it stays below 0.5, the better the long-term prognosis. If the PSA doesn't drop to below 0.5, then statistically you are more likely to have a recurrence of cancer. This is why monitoring the PSA plays an important role. If there is a question about return of the cancer, then you can be followed more closely.

If the PSA starts to go up after radiation therapy, when should I worry?

If I knew this answer, I would be able to tell the future. Much depends on how fast the PSA is going up, how high it is and how long it stayed down after the radiation treatments. The more time it stayed low, the better it is. The slower that it is going up, the better. If it begins to move up rapidly and consistently, then I would be more inclined to start hormone therapy early. Recent studies do show an improved survival advantage for men who have hormone therapy started early rather than late. If your doctor feels the cancer is confined to the prostate, you may be a candidate for salvage prostatectomy, cryotherapy or HIFU.

In my practice, if the PSA keeps increasing (and I check it every four months or so), then I recommend hormone therapy when the PSA goes above 3 or 4. I realize that some experts will say that this is early, but I believe it is easier to control a small amount of cancer early than wait until there is a large volume of cancer. That's when it may be more difficult to stop.

If your PSA is climbing after radiation therapy, stay close to your urologist and follow the PSA level regularly.

If left untreated, how long until the cancer causes problems?

If we had that answer, we would know who should and shouldn't be treated and which treatment to use. That is the dilemma of prostate cancer. Many men will not live long enough for the cancer to be a threat to them, while others may have rapid growth and live long enough to have problems because of the cancer. In general, the less aggressive the cancer, the better your long-term outlook.

What are the treatment options after radiation therapy?

The main option is the addition of hormone therapy. If the PSA starts to rise, then it means that some of the cancer probably wasn't killed by the radiation. It also may mean there was a small bit of cancer outside the field of radiation.

Surgical removal of the prostate after radiation is very difficult with potentially increased risks. This operation is called a *salvage prostatectomy*. Because all the tissues have been radiated, the normal layers between the tissues are usually gone, leaving the tissues all stuck together. This can make it very difficult to remove the prostate gland. Therefore, there is a significant chance of injury to the rectal wall, with a chance of needing a permanent colostomy.

A colostomy is a surgical opening of the large intestine through the skin with drainage of the bowel contents into a bag. This is needed because if the previously radiated rectal wall is damaged, it may not heal well, if at all. The chances of permanent total urinary incontinence are increased following a salvage prostatectomy. There are certain situations where a salvage prostatectomy is a reasonable option when performed by an experienced specialist.

What should the PSA be after hormone therapy?

The lower the PSA goes, the better the result. And the longer it stays low, the more likely it will continue to be low. Hopefully, the PSA will drop to well below 1.0, and maybe as low as 0.1 or even 0.0. The use of hormone therapy alters the normal PSA production, and the PSA test becomes a less accurate tool for monitoring the cancer.

If the PSA goes up after hormone therapy, when should I worry and what are my options?

As with the PSA levels after radiation therapy, much depends on the actual number, how fast it is going up and how long it stayed down on hormone therapy. When it starts to climb above 2 to 5, the disease has progressed to a stage that may be better managed by a urologist or a medical oncologist. I usually ask the patient to at least talk with an oncologist about the options available. You may simply choose to follow the PSA and manage any physical symptoms you experience, or you may choose to try something experimental. Your urologist will either continue caring for you or refer you to the appropriate specialist.

If the PSA begins to go up after surgery or radiation, where are the cancer cells that are causing this increase?

Cancer of the prostate spreads to the lymph nodes and to the bone, but it can also grow into surrounding tissues. The bone scan and CT scan show abnormalities only when the cancer is large enough to produce changes in the bones or to cause fairly significant enlargement or distortion of normal tissues. If the PSA is going up, then we know that the cancer is growing somewhere. The Prostascint scan may add information (explained in Chapter 12).

Is there a role for Proscar or Avodart if the PSA is going up after treatment?

Some specialists have used Proscar or Avodart, occasionally with a drop in the PSA level. No one knows if this treatment actually affects the cancer growth. Some believe it slows cancer progression.

What else can I do to help slow the cancer growth?

If you haven't already done so, I strongly recommend a major change in your diet (described in Chapter 3). At this point you have made a major commitment to your health by undergoing a serious treatment. It only makes sense to follow this step through and pursue a more healthful diet, one high in fruits and vegetables.

Are there any X-rays that are helpful in evaluating where the cancer may have returned after radical prostatectomy?

This is probably the best reason to use the Prostascint scan, again understanding the limitations of the test. Some researchers use an MRI to look for cancer in the area where the prostate used to be.

WILL I NEED ADDITIONAL TREATMENT AFTER RADICAL PROSTATECTOMY?

f the *surgical margins* of your biopsied tissue are found to be positive for cancer, or if there is cancer in the lymph nodes, then the need for additional treatment must be addressed. The surgical margins are the edges of the tissue where the prostate was removed.

Let's address the surgical margins first. Having cancer at the edges of the tissue suggests there may be cancer cells left in the body. When the pathologist looks under the microscope at the tissue, he can see if cancer cells touch the edges of the specimen. If it does, it is labeled as a *positive margin*. A positive surgical margin does not necessarily mean that cancer is left behind.

I recommend checking the PSA level every three months after surgery.

In the past, we sent all of these men with cancer at the margins for a course of additional radiation treatments. Though less radiation may be given after surgery than with regular radiation, it still increases the risks for urinary incontinence and impotence, as well as the standard risks that go along with radiation, including radiation injury to the bladder or rectum.

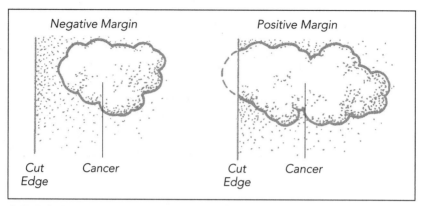

SURGICAL MARGINS. Margins are identified by the pathologist as he or she studies a specimen removed by surgery. A *negative margin* means cancer is not seen at the cut edge and is presumed to be contained within the specimen. A *positive margin* means cancer cells are seen at the cut edge. A positive margin raises the question of whether cancer cells may remain in the body.

I recommend checking the PSA level every three months after surgery. If the level of the PSA begins to increase, then I refer to a radiation therapist for his or her opinion and possible radiation.

After I've had my prostate removed, will I ever need any other treatments for prostate cancer?

Possibly. About one-third of all men will require additional treatments during their lifetime. As nice as it would be to have just one treatment and never have to think about the cancer again, there is always a chance that the cancer may return. You could, indeed, have a significant recurrence of the cancer, requiring further treatment, but your PSA level can also increase without being indicative of anything significant.

What are the options after surgery if additional treatment is needed?

After you've had surgery, the options remaining are radiation and hormone therapy. Radiation will only work if the cancer thought to remain is in the field to be radiated—in other words, *in the pelvis.*

Because of the previous surgery, the dose and length of radiation may be less than if radiation had been used initially. This will depend on your specific situation.

Will I ever need surgery again?

Radical prostatectomy is intended to be the only surgery you should require. You might, however, need to deal with a possible complication such as a lymphatic fluid collection in the abdomen or a scar that might grow at the bladder neck where the urethra was attached to the bladder. Fortunately, these complications tend to be fairly rare and are usually treated in minor outpatient procedures.

The risks of adding on radiation treatment include increased urinary incontinence and impotence, as well as irritation and injury to the bladder or rectal wall.

Does the amount of tumor at the margin make a difference?
Yes. If there is only a small speck of tumor at the margin, then we would probably just follow you conservatively with a PSA test on a regular basis.

However, if there is a large amount of cancer at the cut edge, suggesting a significant amount of tumor may be left behind, then we would probably recommend radiation once you have recovered from the surgery. Even with a significant positive margin, 30% to 50% of men do not have a recurrence of the cancer. The margins of most concern are along the back wall (posterior) of the prostate. Positive margins at the apex or along the side (laterally) are less significant.

What about hormone therapy?
Hormone therapy is used when it is believed that additional treatment is needed and either radiation alone won't take care of the problem (if the cancer is outside the pelvis) or a more conservative, less risky treatment is believed best.

DO I NEED CHEMOTHERAPY?

36

C hemotherapy is not a main treatment choice for prostate cancer, although it is routinely used for treatment of other types of cancer. The other treatments already discussed are more effective. However, when the cancer continues to grow and other treatments have been tried, we often turn to chemotherapy to try to slow and control the cancer growth.

I don't think any chemotherapy doctors, or *oncologists*, will tell you they hope for a cure with chemotherapy. Rather, the goal with chemotherapy is to stop or at least slow the cancer. Even in the best of hands, chemotherapy may work in 20% to 40% of the men who receive it. How long it works is variable. And how well it works is unpredictable.

According to prostate cancer expert Dr. Frederick Ahmann at the Arizona Cancer Center, the big question with chemotherapy is whether its possible benefit outweighs its probable side effects. The treatment may add only a few months to your life span, and you may spend those months weak and nauseated. Then again, it may provide excellent control for months to years with a normal life span and good quality of life. You must

> *The big question with chemotherapy is whether its possible benefit outweighs its probable side effects.*

294

decide if it is worth the effort and expense, both financially and emotionally.

I know of one patient who died as a result of chemotherapy. On the other hand, there are patients who seem to tolerate chemotherapy without difficulty and have dramatic benefits.

There are different types of chemotherapy. A number of them may hold some promise for treating prostate cancer. Each type of cancer is treated with different chemical agents at different doses. The goal is to kill fast-growing cancer cells with the medication. Each chemotherapy medication functions individually and in combination to kill cancer cells through specific pathways, such as blocking angiogenesis so the cancer cells can't grow or spread. Others work by freezing the cancer cells at particular points in their growth cycle, while others simply restart the normal programmed cell death (apoptosis) so the cells begin to die as they were designed to do. Some chemotherapy agents restore the microtubule environment within the cell, which allows the cells to communicate again with neighboring cells and bring back the growth patterns and limitations seen in normal cells. Remember that each cancer is different, each person is different and each person's cancer responds differently to these medications. Though many may think there is a minimal role for chemo, I have seen some amazing results with long-term survival!

Are there experimental chemotherapy drugs available?
In many communities, you may be eligible for experimental agents as part of research treatment plans, or protocols, where a medication is being tried. Sometimes these experimental drugs don't work. Occasionally they provide good results.

Docetaxel

Docetaxel is an exciting and very promising chemotherapy medication that restores the intracellular architecture of the cancer cells, stabilizes the microtubules and may block angiogenesis (promotion of abnormal and new blood vessels). Dr. Ahmann is very optimistic about potential benefits of docetaxel. Docetaxel can be used alone or in combination with other medications. In addition, docetaxel leads to cell-cycle arrest (stopping the cancer cells from

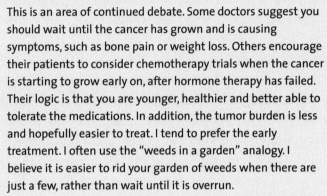

When should I start chemotherapy?

This is an area of continued debate. Some doctors suggest you should wait until the cancer has grown and is causing symptoms, such as bone pain or weight loss. Others encourage their patients to consider chemotherapy trials when the cancer is starting to grow early on, after hormone therapy has failed. Their logic is that you are younger, healthier and better able to tolerate the medications. In addition, the tumor burden is less and hopefully easier to treat. I tend to prefer the early treatment. I often use the "weeds in a garden" analogy. I believe it is easier to rid your garden of weeds when there are just a few, rather than wait until it is overrun.

During chemotherapy treatments, we may stop the standard hormone blockade, while at other times it is continued. Talk to your doctor. If one approach doesn't work for you, then perhaps it is time to try another.

growing) at a point in the cycle where the cancer cell is more sensitive to the killing effect of radiation.

Thalidomide

This medication has been shown to have some definite benefits in treating advanced prostate cancer. Thalidomide is an antiangiogenesis medication that prevents the cancer from stimulating new blood vessels.

COX$_2$ Inhibitors

Cancer cells can be blocked from creating new blood vessel growth (angiogenesis) and stimulated to die (apoptosis) using COX$_2$ inhibitors. Relatively new on the market as anti-inflammation medications for arthritis, cyclooxygenase-2 inhibitors (COX$_2$ inhibitors) such as Celebrex (celecoxib) are being used to enhance the effectiveness of chemotherapy.

Immune Therapy

There are many exciting advances and study protocols stimulating the body's own immune system to attack and kill prostate cancer cells. Some involve using altered viruses to destroy the cancer.

Ketaconozole and Nizoral

These medications are routinely used to treat fungal infections. They were always known to block the body's ability to produce male hormones. Urologists and medical oncologists have started using ketaconozole or Nizoral to treat prostate cancer that has failed standard hormone therapy. Although these medications do not work for everyone, many men have a positive response.

The main side effect is possible but unlikely serious liver damage, so it is important to check blood tests of liver function on a regular basis.

DES

Although infrequently used, DES, discussed in Chapter 24, can be given in higher doses to treat advanced prostate cancer. DES can be very effective, providing excellent control of the cancer growth through a number of mechanisms. The main danger with a high dose of DES is the risk of blood clots, heart attacks and strokes. For this reason, men are often put on blood thinners, such as Coumadin, at the same time. I have seen very impressive responses to high-dose DES therapy.

Hydrocortisone and Mitoxantrone

This is a combination therapy of a steroid, hydrocortisone, and a standard chemotherapy drug, Mitoxantrone. Some studies have shown very good results. This combination is very well tolerated, with few side effects. Studies suggest that the majority of the benefits may come from the hydrocortisone. Many researchers prefer the combination. Others prefer prednisone. This combination is a reasonable therapy to discuss with your doctor.

TNP 470

This is a chemical formulation of a natural substance extracted from a fungus, which blocks angiogenesis of the growing prostate cancer cells.

Endostatin

This protein has also been shown to block angiogenesis.

2ME (methoxyestradiol)

This natural breakdown product of the female hormone estrogen is a potent blocker of tumor angiogenesis and stimulates apoptosis.

Exisulind (sulindac sulfone)

Exisulind is a powerful anti-inflammatory medication that has been shown to kill prostate cancer cells and induce apoptosis, especially when used with other anticancer medications.

Alternative, Complementary and Integrative Options

Some men with advanced disease will turn to nontraditional options and perhaps decline chemotherapy. The benefits and risks of nontraditional approaches are reviewed in Chapter 26. Some nontraditional options may have actual benefits. Many don't and are just a way to take advantage of your panic and vulnerability.

To those who urge you to have nontraditional treatment, ask the same questions you would of any standard treatment. Do your research and know what you're getting into. Many times these treatments are a pure waste of money. I have seen many situations in which patients opted for natural cures, only to realize too late that they had spent many thousands of dollars and wasted months or years with no help. These unproven treatments are often scams that keep you from taking proven and effective therapies. Be skeptical. If it sounds too good to be true, it usually is.

Side Effects

Side effects are always the big concern any time the word "chemotherapy" is heard. Potential side effects vary from drug to drug and person to person. Some side effects are minimal, while others can be quite severe or even fatal.

Your oncologist can tell you specifically which chemotherapy options are best for you, whether or not you are a candidate for any experimental drugs or research protocols and what possible side effects you might expect.

RESEARCH STUDIES— LOOKING FOR NEW CURES

37

A number of exciting new prostate cancer treatments will be available in the near future. Almost all major advances in medicine are first tested in experimental studies. Men with prostate cancer may be able to benefit from experimental treatments at a university or community hospital. But it is important to be aware of the risks as well as the possible benefits of subjecting yourself to medical research studies.

Don't university hospitals have research studies that I might want to join or participate in?

Yes, most advances in cancer research and treatment do come out of academic teaching centers. This occurs because researchers are able to try new, untested procedures and medication programs. Some of the procedures and medications will not work, but others will.

Many patients will be able to get an otherwise unavailable treatment that may help, while other patients get a standard and possibly less effective treatment. Most often, researchers compare what they hope to be a better treatment with one that is already proven to be effective. Enrolling in a clinical study will be helpful for the good of society and future patients with a similar problem. This system is how researchers learn what will and will not work in medicine.

How will they decide which treatments are best for me?

In the university teaching-center environment, doctors have a number of treatment plans, called *research protocols*, available. The doctors look at your medical situation and try to determine which protocol would be the best fit.

What are some questions to ask before becoming a patient in a research study?

Talk with the doctors and ask questions about the treatments to be studied. What specifically is the study trying to prove? Find out how long the study has been under way and if any preliminary results are available.

Ask how long you will be on the treatment plan. What kind of follow-up, tests and procedures will be needed? How often do you have to come back for tests? Who will do these tests and who will pay for them? Who will pay for the medications, surgery, radiation and other procedures?

If there is a complication, who will pay for those costs and provide the care? Can you leave anytime if you're not happy? What are the risks of entering this trial as compared with standard therapy? Who is sponsoring (paying for) the study? How will you be monitored?

Can I be involved in these same experimental studies in the private sector, outside of a university setting?

Yes, you should be able to. Most communities have a number of private-practice cancer specialists who are participants in the same research trials.

?

In a research study, can I decide what treatment I want for me?

No, you usually have to agree to be randomized, which means you will be randomly assigned by a computer to one treatment or another. Using this method, the research results will more accurately reflect the benefits or disadvantages of a specific treatment, rather than the patient's choices.

What if I'm not happy with the treatment choice that I'm assigned to?
You may have the option to quit, depending on the study. You shouldn't enter into a research study unless you are willing to accept any of the treatments being analyzed. It's not fair to the people trying to run the study to invest the time and effort only to have people drop out because they don't like the assigned treatment.

Could I be assigned to a treatment that is potentially dangerous?
This is always possible because the studies often are looking at unproven therapies that are effective in the lab. You should clearly understand what the study is trying to prove and the pros and cons of each of the treatment options.

How do I find out about research studies on prostate cancer?
Contact a regional cancer-research center.

What is a clinical trial?
This is the testing of a new drug in humans. Phase I evaluates the drug's safety. Phase II evaluates the drug's effectiveness. Phase III is a large-scale evaluation of the safety and effectiveness before it is approved for general use.

Future Areas of Research

Some new areas of research are immune stimulation, vaccines, early detection, understanding early cancer growth and spread, and genetic factors.

IMMUNE STIMULATION AND VACCINES

These immune cells are removed from the blood stream, activated to seek out and destroy a specific target, and then placed back in the body. The ideal treatment for a cancer would be to stimulate your own body's immune system to fight off and kill the cancer. This is being done in bladder-cancer treatment. Studies are under way throughout the world.

Some research may identify a vaccine that can locate and kill prostate-cancer cells. This may be most useful after radical surgery to find and kill any cells that remain.

EARLY DETECTION

The ideal time to detect a prostate cancer is when it is still confined to the prostate gland and easy to cure. While the PSA blood test is good, it still is far from perfect.

Research is under way on new modifications and variations to the PSA test that may pick up advanced cancer that has spread. Accurate detection of cancer outside the prostate helps us select the most appropriate treatment and avoid unnecessary procedures.

There are some new studies looking at various aspects of the cancer cells themselves, the number of blood vessels around the cancer, associated proteins and the cancer's DNA to determine if they can accurately predict the cancer's behavior. There are some exciting new advances in treatment, including hyperthermia, gamma interferon, immunization against the cancer cells and genetically altering the tumors with "designer" viruses. Designer viruses are altered to infect the cancer cells and "trick" them into dying.

EARLY CANCER GROWTH AND SPREAD

Researchers are investigating what stimulates angiogenesis, the growth of new blood vessels that supply tiny cancers with nutrients, allowing them to grow larger. If a chemical could be identified that stimulates this blood-vessel growth, perhaps that chemical could be blocked so no cancer could ever grow beyond just a few cells in size.

Scientists are looking at why cancer cells can penetrate into blood vessels and then break loose and spread. If the blood vessels could become more resistant to cancer-cell penetration with a treatment, maybe the cancers could be prevented from spreading.

There are studies trying to identify which substances encourage cancer cells to grow elsewhere in the body. This, too, could lead to a treatment to keep cancers from spreading.

GENETIC RESEARCH

Genetics, the study of heredity and how our genes and diseases are related, is a promising field in which researchers are trying to identify which genes are responsible for development of cancer. Clearly, for some men, genes play a role in their cancer growth. Researchers are looking at "suicide gene" therapy to force cancers to die.

Studies are looking at genetic markers that may suggest higher vulnerability to developing prostate cancer. These abnormal spots in the DNA can be passed on to children, which may explain why some prostate cancers can run in families and are considered hereditary prostate cancer. The more of these abnormal markers you have, the higher your risk.

OTHER QUESTIONS

Are there some genes that somehow enable environmental factors to stimulate prostate cancer to grow?

Could this be how a high-fat diet encourages prostate cancer to develop?

Do some men have certain genes that suppress prostate cancer development?

Can these protective genes be inactivated by diet or the environment, enabling prostate cancer to grow?

Are there certain enzymes in the body that, when blocked by a genetic change, enable cancers to grow?

We don't know the answers to these questions. But research is under way around the world to try to solve these puzzles about the origin of not only prostate cancer, but all cancers.

I am always amazed by the dedication and commitment of many tens of thousands of researchers and scientists to find the answers to these and other questions, all with the goal of preventing and curing prostate cancer. Next time you drive by a research lab or hospital late one night, look up and see how many lights are still on—doctors, scientists and researchers working for you and your children.

WHEN ALL TREATMENTS FAIL

38

A
ll the best standard treatments and therapies for prostate disease sometimes just don't work, and the cancer may continue to grow. When this happens, there are questions that most doctors and health-care providers don't feel comfortable answering.

Please, before you read this chapter, understand that it addresses death from prostate cancer, and rather bluntly at that. Some men have told me that this chapter upset them. Others thanked me for dealing with this otherwise taboo subject.

The following questions and answers are very matter-of-fact. You should read this chapter only if you *really* want to know the answers. I have found that some men and their wives would rather not know this information.

It is provided here because I believe it is important for you to have access to this information if you want to know the worst-case scenarios. At some point, it may become clear what is inevitably around the turn. As a friend of mine once said, "No one gets out of here alive." We all have to go sometime. For the patient whose cancer defies treatment and continues to grow, I hope we can help make this transition more tolerable for him and his family.

> *If the cancer continues to grow, how long will I live?*
>
> **?**
>
> This depends on how advanced the cancer is. In the worst situations, you may have just a few months, or you may have many years or more. There is no possible way to predict for an individual how long he will survive with the cancer growing. There are occasions when a patient will have rapid growth of the cancer despite everything we do.
>
> At the other extreme, it is quite common for many men to live years longer than was predicted. Some men with advanced disease can be alive and well a decade later. In my years traveling and speaking to support groups, I have met many men who outlived doctors who had predicted their quick death.

How do we know that the cancer has come back?
Usually the PSA level will continue to rise. The PSA can go up into the hundreds and even into the thousands. Sometimes an irregularity can be felt on rectal examination. Some men complain of vague aches or pains, or weakness and fatigue that suggest the cancer may have spread.

Do I need additional X-rays or tests?
A repeat bone scan, CT scan or X-ray may be performed to learn if and where the cancer has returned.

Do I need to have a repeat biopsy?
Not usually. Your doctors usually will have a fairly accurate idea what the problem is. If there are any questions about the source of a lesion, lump or abnormality, a repeat biopsy may be necessary.

How fast can the cancer grow?
This is highly variable and can even fluctuate within a single person. For many men the cancer can take many years to become significant. Even then, it can grow so slowly that for selected patients, treatment may be indefinitely postponed.

For other men, however, the cancer can grow rapidly, sometimes killing the person in a matter of months from the time of diagnosis. Most often, even in the most advanced cancers, the growth may take many months or even a few years.

What are the expected symptoms as the cancer grows?
In advanced cases, when all standard treatments fail, you might notice increasing fatigue, gradual weight loss, weakness, depression, changing aches and pain and loss of appetite.

Can anything be done to help my appetite?
Sometimes treatment with steroids, such as oral prednisone, can improve your appetite and give you a feeling of well-being.

How will the cancer actually kill me if we can't control it?
Most cancers kill by growing and spreading to vital organs in the body, overloading and preventing normal organ function. Prostate cancer doesn't seem to work this way. Prostate cancer will continue to grow and increase in volume in your lymph nodes and in the bone marrow.

It appears that prostate cancer in large volumes releases toxic substances into the bloodstream. These substances account for many of the symptoms seen with advanced prostate cancer. These toxic substances were originally part of normal prostatic secretions. However, in the bloodstream they can cause loss of appetite, fatigue and gradual wasting, ultimately leading to death.

What else can happen as the cancer grows?
Your blood counts may go down, making you anemic, as the tissues of the bone marrow that produce blood are replaced by cancer. You may feel weak and fatigued. The bones may become weakened and brittle, and it is possible that you could experience sudden fractures. This is most common in weight-bearing bones, such as in the hips and top of the legs.

Sometimes a tumor in the spine can enlarge and squeeze the spinal cord, causing numbness or weakness in the legs. This is a true emergency and needs immediate attention to prevent you from becoming paralyzed!

Will I be in pain?

Many times, yes. Pain depends on *exactly where* the cancer has spread and *how much* cancer you have in your body. If the cancer has spread to the bones, this often can result in quite a lot of pain. If the cancer is growing in the lymph nodes, this usually does not cause pain unless the enlarged nodes are compressing and squeezing critical areas, such as nerves or the ureters that drain urine from the kidneys.

Can the pain be controlled?

For most men, usually. Doctors have access to a large number of long-acting and powerful pain medications and narcotics to help control severe pain. I often use a combination of medications to allow for the most accurate control of pain.

If the pain becomes very severe, then radiation treatments to the painful bone will sometimes block any pain. These treatments also serve to strengthen the bone and prevent any break. I often ask pain specialists (usually an anesthesiologist who specializes in pain management) to see if they can block the pain with specialized pain medications and long-acting injections.

Are there any treatments to reduce pain from cancer that has spread to the bone?

Yes. A radioactive substance can be injected into the veins to kill cancer cells in the bone. An example of this new type of medication is strontium 89, available under the brand name Metastron. The medication costs $12,000 for the first treatment and then $6,000 for each additional treatment.

How effective is this type of treatment?

The results vary from person to person, but in general up to 70% of men with severe pain in the bones not helped by routine pain medication will describe some improvement, often within a few weeks. Although the degree of pain control is unpredictable, some men may even have total relief from bone pain. How long the benefits last is also quite variable.

Are there any side effects to this new medication?
Occasionally, the medication can interfere with the normal production of blood. To watch for this, you will need to have blood counts checked on a regular basis after the treatment. This side effect can be severe and require transfusions.

If the bone pain goes away, can the treatment be repeated if the pain comes back?
Yes. If you have good results with your first treatment, you can have an additional treatment or two, no sooner than every six months.

Are there any ways of controlling pain without medications?
Yes. Methods include *biofeedback, relaxation techniques, meditation, mental imagery, distraction, skin stimulation* and *massage.* Some men find relief with acupuncture and acupressure, hypnosis and electrical nerve stimulators. Before you start any of these procedures, check with your doctor, because some may cause problems.

How can I learn more about these options?
One of the best sources is the pamphlet *Questions and Answers About Pain Control,* published by and available from the American Cancer Society. Pain clinics often have literature and books.

How does kidney failure kill a person?
Ordinarily, the kidneys filter the blood and remove toxic wastes, which are then excreted in the urine. If the kidneys are blocked by the cancer as it squeezes the ureters shut, then the waste products will slowly build up in your system. At some point, you may experience increasing fatigue, weakness, a loss of appetite and occasionally itching. The itching is from the accumulation of waste products in the tissues. Left untreated, you would gradually become weaker and weaker. Then you would quietly slip into a coma and die peacefully.

How long does it take to die from kidney failure?
This is highly variable and can take weeks, many months or longer. Sometimes there can be severe but not total obstruction, with the kidneys still

filtering toxic wastes just enough to keep you alive but still with significant kidney failure. This can last indefinitely.

What can be done if I have kidney failure?

The big question is not how we address kidney failure but rather should we even try to solve this problem. If the cancer is so significant as to cause kidney failure from blockage, then relieving the blockage of the kidneys may just prolong your life even when death is just around the corner.

If you do decide to treat the kidney obstruction, the main approach is to place a small catheter, called a *nephrostomy tube*, into the kidney through the skin on your side. This tube drains into a small bag, which has to be periodically emptied. Nephrostomy tubes are usually placed by radiologists or urologists in an outpatient procedure using just a local anesthesia.

Another way to place these drainage tubes is to pass small catheters, called *ureteral stents*, up the ureter through the penis, usually under anesthesia. With this technique, it is sometimes impossible to pass the tube up to the kidney. Then you must have the tubes placed by a radiologist through the skin.

Is kidney failure a bad way to die?

No. Death in this manner is considered one of the least unpleasant ways to die. Most men with kidney failure complain that they have lost their appetite, or they feel weak or fatigued or itchy. Gradually, you become weaker and weaker, simply fading into a coma, followed by death.

What's the advisability of trying an alternative or herbal "last-ditch" treatment?

There will always be those who prey on desperate men and women who are willing to try anything at any price to stop the cancer from growing.

In my practice, I don't believe I should deny patients the option to seek out alternative choices. I try to encourage patients to pursue alternative treatments *in addition* to known and accepted options, not *instead* of those standard treatments. I do ask patients to be as critical and challenging to the alternative health-care provider as they were of their regular doctor.

What is hospice?

This can be a facility where terminally ill patients can go near the end of their lives for supportive care while they die. It is a place where nurses, doctors and support staff are all specifically trained to attend to the special needs of the dying patient. Hospice can also be in your own home with the same "visiting" services. Hospice is usually a positive and caring experience for everyone involved, and allows for your passing with grace, respect and dignity.

I have had several patients who accept as fact the claims and recommendations made by an acquaintance who promotes unheard-of herbal therapy or teaches a bizarre diet for cancer. Yet these same accepting patients routinely challenge me to prove with extensive facts, research studies and documentation the benefits of any treatment that I suggest.

What should I watch out for if I'm considering alternative treatments?
Beware of testimonial-style marketing, where a small number of men and women claim to have had a miraculous recovery with a treatment.

If it looks easy, with results almost *too good to be true*, it usually is. If it is very expensive, watch out. Many of these treatments require cash up front. This should make you very suspicious.

Watch out if this elaborate and expensive treatment is completed in just a weekend, especially if it is in a country with few limitations on unproven treatments.

What about hospice as the cancer progresses?
Hospice care may be reasonable for advanced stages of cancer. Hospice nurses can provide more pain control, nutritional care and attention to the problems that can develop with a dying patient. Some communities and facilities have home hospice services where a trained nurse or aide comes to the home to

help care for a terminally ill person. Hospice also provides important emotional and psychological support for everyone involved.

How do I prepare for my death?

Though this is difficult to think about, it is best to look at what aspects of your life you have control over. Make needed arrangements so that your wife or family won't be burdened after your death. Make sure the house, the cars, any investments, business accounts and credit cards are all in good legal order so that your wife or family will not face difficult legal obstacles. Set up trusts. Talk to an attorney or financial adviser.

Talk to your friends. Visit family. Spend time with those you care about. As difficult as this transition is for you, it is probably much harder for your wife and children. Be supportive and comforting.

What about my legal concerns?

The American Cancer Society has an excellent pamphlet on what should be addressed by you regarding legal questions, business, taxes and loans. A brief list of things to organize includes:

- Life insurance
- Retirement plan
- Title to any assets that you have
- Property
- Bank accounts
- Collections (debts owed to you)
- Safe deposit boxes
- Vehicle deeds
- Will

For each of these items you should record account numbers, addresses, phone numbers, contact people and the locations of important keys and papers.

What about a "living will"?

This is very important to guarantee that no measures are taken *against your wishes* simply to sustain your life. You should talk to your doctor or lawyer about a living will, and you should sign a general "durable power of attorney" and a "medical durable power of attorney" to give your family or friends the necessary authority to make decisions for you. You may want to establish a possible guardian or conservator or put together a "living trust."

What should I do with my living will and medical power of attorney forms?

It is very important that you make copies and deliver them to your doctors to file with your records. Keep the original with you at home. If you go to the hospital, bring a copy with you *every time*. Even if you brought one with you to the hospital previously, it may be "lost" somewhere in medical records. It may not be readily accessible when you need it in an emergency, so bring your own copy.

SUPPORT GROUPS AND RESOURCES

39

S upport groups can play an important role in helping you decide which treatments to consider, which doctors to see, perhaps even which ones to avoid. Groups can provide a comfortable environment where you can share your deepest fears or concerns with men who have experienced what you are going through.

Support groups provide strategies for coping with your cancer and any hurdles that may come up.

A recent study suggested that women who attended breast-cancer support groups survived longer than those women who didn't. This raises the point of just how important your mental and emotional health are in dealing with cancer. Perhaps there's more to the cure than surgery or radiation.

Perhaps there's more to the cure than surgery or radiation.

Support groups provide camaraderie and bonding with other men who understand what no one else can. I strongly suggest that patients seek out a support group in the community. Even if you don't want to talk, just listening will help.

What happens at support group meetings?

There are different types of groups. Their meetings may vary widely in focus and purpose. Some groups are purely informational, with visiting speakers on new advances and treatment options, dietary recommendations, new medications and how to cope with the changes in your life. Other meetings may consist of simply sharing thoughts, fears and concerns. Some groups have formal leaders, while others may just have a freestyle format. The goal is to increase your level of knowledge and to give you back that feeling of control that is lost with the unknown of cancer disease.

Why should I go to a group and remind myself of what I've got and what may happen to me in the future?

These groups aren't intended to overwhelm you and occupy all your waking thoughts. In fact, you might come to realize it's okay to have cancer but that it shouldn't be the focus of your life. Even in the worst-case scenarios, most men will have years ahead of them before they even have to address their mortality. You should at least go and give it a try.

Is it true that most men who go to support groups are the ones who are really sick and are looking for some new treatment?

There's some truth to this. Men who are having continued problems are probably more likely to attend support-group meetings to share experiences

How do I find a support group in my area?

First ask your urologist. He may know of some in or near your community. If you are unable to locate one, call your local chapter of the American Cancer Society. You also can call the number for the international support group US-TOO (see the next section on resources in this chapter) to see if there is a group nearby. Talk to your friends. If there is a group in your community, you should be able to locate it by following these suggestions.

and learn what's new. But quite often there will be a few men who were just recently diagnosed with prostate cancer. They are looking for some advice and guidance. It is quite helpful to be there to tell someone what it's like, that the surgery really isn't so scary or that the radiation is well tolerated. Most importantly, they need to hear that yes, there is a light at the end of the tunnel.

Resources

Following is a list of some of the resources that are available to you and your family. Most are unbiased, although a few may have their own preferences for therapy. Some are established by pharmaceutical or manufacturing companies to help promote their own products. I have had a few patients who made important decisions regarding their care because of information they received from some of these sources.

Information from these sources, like this book, should serve as a foundation of knowledge for you to use when you talk with your doctors about your care. This book is not intended to make a decision for you. Each person is different from everyone else. What may look good on paper may actually not be best for you.

AMERICAN CANCER SOCIETY

The American Cancer Society is a voluntary health organization that offers a wide variety of services and literature to patients and their families at no charge. Literature is available on all cancers, nutrition, stress and anxiety, plus legal and financial planning. Some chapters provide information regarding transportation (or can refer you) if needed, support groups and a range of other helpful services locally. The society is also involved in funding scientific research and community education. You can check with your local chapter (look on the Internet and in the white pages), or contact the national office:

Call: 1-800-227-2345
Write: American Cancer Society
1599 Clifton Rd. NE
Atlanta, GA 30329-4251
Website: www.cancer.org

AVA FOUNDATION

Foundation sponsored by the American Urologic Association to provide urologic education, research and outreach.

Call: 1-800-828-7866
Write: 1000 Corporate Blvd.
Linthicum Heights, MD 21090
Website: www.avafoundation.org

AMERICAN RED CROSS

Resources available to train relatives in home nursing care and first aid.

Call: Your local chapter (see white pages) or 1-202-737-8300
Write: American Red Cross
430 17th St. NW
Washington, DC 20006
Website: www.redcross.org

BOARD CERTIFICATION

To find out if your doctor is board-certified, you can call this number or check in the *Directory of Medical Specialists*, which should be available at most libraries. Check to make sure the volume you are looking at is current.

Call: 1-866-275-2267 (United States)
1-613-730-8177 (Canada)
Website: www.certifieddoctor.org
www.certifacts.org or www.abms.org

CANADIAN CANCER SOCIETY

This is the sister organization of the American Cancer Society, providing the same resources, information, literature and community support services for individuals with cancer.

Call: 1-416-961-7223
Write: Canadian Cancer Society
10 Alcorn Ave., Ste. 200
Toronto, ON M4V 3B1
Canada
Website: www.cancer.ca

CANCER CARE INC.

Part of the National Cancer Foundation, the Prostate Cancer Education Council will provide information and counseling to patients and families, as well as assistance for nonmedical expenses. Many services are for the greater New York area, but information is available nationwide.

Call: 1-800-813-4673
Write: Cancer Care Inc.
275 Seventh Ave.
New York, NY 10001
Website: www.cancercare.org

GEDDINGS OSBON FOUNDATION

Information and a booklet on impotence, primarily focusing on vacuum erection devices, but reviewing all options.

Call: 1-800-433-4215
Write: Geddings Osbon Foundation
P.O. Box 1593
Augusta, GA 30903-1593
Website: www.impotence.org

INSTITUTE FOR UROLOGIC EXCELLENCE

Steven K. Wilson, M.D., World's Leading Penile Prosthesis Expert
Call: 1-760-342-6657
Write: 81-719 Dr. Carreon Blvd., Pod C
Indio, CA 92201-5518
Website: www.visitiue.com

NATIONAL ASSOCIATION FOR CONTINENCE

A nonprofit organization that provides information on urinary incontinence.
Call: 1-800-BLADDER
Write: National Association for Continence
P.O. Box 8310
Spartanburg, SC 29305
Website: www.nafc.org

NATIONAL CANCER INSTITUTE (NCI)

The NCI provides written material and information on a variety of cancer-related topics, and it makes referrals to local and regional cancer-treatment centers.

Call: The Cancer Information Service at 1-800-4-CANCER
(1-800-422-6237)
Write: Office of Cancer Communications
National Cancer Institute
Building 31, Room 10A16
Bethesda, MD 20892
Website: www.nci.nih.gov

NATIONAL COALITION FOR CANCER SURVIVORSHIP

This is a network of survivors and related organizations that can provide information regarding local and regional support groups. The coalition works for cancer survivors as an advocate in the workplace, especially regarding discrimination.

Call: 1-888-650-9127
Write: National Coalition for Cancer Survivorship
1010 Wayne Ave., 5th Floor
Silver Springs, MD 20910
Website: www.canceradvocacy.org

PATIENT ADVOCATES FOR ADVANCED CANCER TREATMENTS (PAACT)

This is a clearinghouse for information on new and nonsurgical cancer treatments.

Call: 1-616-453-1477
Fax: 1-616-453-1846
Write: PAACT
P.O. Box 141695
Grand Rapids, MI 49514-1695
Website: www.paactusa.org

PROSTATE CANCER AWARENESS NETWORK

This is one of the leading nationwide prostate-cancer support networks, pursuing government advocacy issues, financing research and focusing on increasing public awareness of prostate cancer.

    Call: 1-800-828-7866
    Write: Prostate Cancer Support Group
    300 W. Pratt St., Ste. 401
    Baltimore, MD 21201

PROSTATE CANCER RESEARCH INSTITUTE

This is a nonprofit research organization dedicated to education, prevention and treatment of prostate cancer.

    Call: 1-310-743-2110
    Write: Prostate Cancer Research Institute
    4676 Admiralty Way, Ste. 103
    Marina del Rey, CA 90292
    Website: www.prostate-cancer.org

PROSTATE FORUM

The excellent monthly newsletter by Dr. Charles "Snuffy" Myers on nutrition and prostate cancer. One of the best if you are serious about understanding how your diet affects prostate cancer and treatment.

    Call: 1-800-305-2432
    Write: Prostate Forum
    P.O. Box 6696
    Charlottesville, VA 22906
    Website: www.prostateforum.com

SEX INFORMATION AND EDUCATION COUNCIL OF THE UNITED STATES

Provides literature on sexuality and illness.

    Call: 1-212-819-9770
    Write: Sex Information and Education Council of the United States
    90 John St., Ste. 704
    New York, NY 10038
    Website: www.siecus.org

THE SIMON FOUNDATION

An educational service providing information on urinary incontinence and treatment options.

    Call: 1-800-23-SIMON (1-800-237-4666)
    Write: The Simon Foundation
    P.O. Box 835
    Wilmette, IL 60091
    Website: www.simonfoundation.org

US-TOO PROSTATE CANCER SURVIVOR SUPPORT GROUPS

One of the largest patient-organized support groups that focuses on survivor support and offers fellowship and counseling.

    Call: 1-800-808-7866
    Write: US-TOO
    5003 Fairview Ave.
    Downers Grove, IL 60515
    Website: www.ustoo.org

Newsletters

HARVARD HEALTH LETTER

    164 Longwood Ave.
    Boston, MA 02115
    Monthly/$32.00 per year
    1-800-829-9045
    www.health.harvard.edu

JOHNS HOPKINS MEDICAL LETTER: HEALTH AFTER 50

    Medical Association
    632 Broadway
    New York, NY 10012-2614
    Monthly/$28.00 per year or $24.00 per year through Internet
    1-800-829-0422
    www.hopkinsafter50.com

MAYO CLINIC HEALTH LETTER

Mayo Foundation for Medical Education and Research
200 First St. NW
Rochester, MN 55905
Monthly/$27.00 per year
1-800-333-9037
www.mayohealth.org

PROSTATE FORUM

P.O. Box 6696
Charlottesville, VA 22906
Monthly/$84.00 per year
1-800-305-2432
www.prostateforum.com

TUFTS UNIVERSITY HEALTH & NUTRITION LETTER

53 Park Place
New York, NY 10007
Monthly/$28.00 per year
1-800-274-7581
www.healthletter.tufts.edu

UNIVERSITY OF CALIFORNIA AT BERKELEY WELLNESS LETTER

Prince Street Station
P.O. Box 412
New York, NY 10012-0007
Monthly/$28.00 per year
1-800-829-9170
www.berkeleywellness.com

Books

If you want to know more than most urologists about prostate cancer as well as new and cutting-edge treatment options. I strongly suggest this book.

Strum, Stephen B., and Donna Pogliano. *The Primer on Prostate Cancer: The Empowered Patient's Guide.* Fort Lauderdale, FL: Life Extension Media, 2002.

Available from Amazon at www.amazon.com, LEF (Life Extension Foundation) at www.lefprostate.org or 1-866-820-7457, Us Too at www.ustoo.com or 1-317-558-4858 or 1-800-808-7866, or PCRI (Prostate Cancer Research Institute) at www.pcri.org or 310-743-2110.

Website

This is an excellent resource on prostate cancer, and it's one of my favorites: http://prostatecancerinfolink.net.

GLOSSARY

Terms used in this glossary may not be used elsewhere in the book, but they may be used by your doctor or in other literature that you read regarding prostate disease.

A

abdomen. Lower part of the torso that contains the intestines, liver, stomach and spleen.

abdominal aortic aneurysm. Abnormal swelling and weakening of the large artery that takes blood from the heart to the rest of the body.

acid phosphatase. Substance made in the prostate.

adenocarcinoma. Cancer made of abnormal gland cells from the lining of an organ. Most prostate cancers are adenocarcinomas.

adjuvant therapy. Addition of radiation, hormone therapy or chemotherapy after surgery.

adjuvant treatment. Treatment added to the main surgical treatment.

adrenal glands. Glands located above each kidney. They produce several kinds of hormones, including sex hormones.

age-adjusted. Looking at a lab result as it relates to a person's age.

alkaline phosphatase. Enzyme produced in the liver and bones that is used to help determine whether a prostate cancer has spread to the bones.

anaphylactic reaction. Sudden and life-threatening reaction to a substance or medication.

androgen blockade. Blockage of the male hormones called *androgens*.

androgens. A hormonal substance necessary for the development and functioning of the male sex organs and male sexual characteristics, such as deep voice and facial hair.

anesthesia. Using a medication or substance to eliminate or block pain, as during a surgical procedure.

anterior. Front of an organ or structure.

antiandrogen. Medication that reduces or eliminates the presence or activity of androgens in the body.

antibiotic. A medication used to kill germs that can cause infection.

anti-inflammatory. Medication that reduces pain, swelling, redness and irritation from injury, surgery or infection.

anus. The opening of the rectum.

apex. Tip of the prostate, farthest away from the bladder.

artificial urinary sphincter. Surgically implanted prosthetic device that compresses the urethra and reduces urine leakage.

aspiration. Removal of fluid or tissue by using suction, usually through a fine needle.

atypia. Suspicious changes on biopsy highly suggestive of cancer.

autologous transfusions. Using a person's own blood for transfusion during surgery.

B

bacteria. One-celled microscopic organisms that can cause infection under certain conditions.

balloon dilation. An abandoned technique used in the past to stretch open the prostate, with the goal of improving urine flow.

base. Wide part of the prostate adjacent to the bladder.

benign. A growth that is not cancerous.

beta carotene. A nutrient found in vegetables; important for normal health.

bicalutamide. Generic name for *Casodex,* an antiandrogen.

bilateral. Both sides, as in *bilateral orchiectomy.*

biopsy. Removal of small samples of tissue for microscopic examination to see whether cancer is present.

bladder. Organ in which urine is stored before it is discharged from the body.

bladder neck. Circular muscle fibers that come together like a funnel where the bladder opens into the prostate.

bladder spasms. Painful squeezing of the bladder in response to irritation or injury.

blood clot. Thickening of blood to form a solid mass similar to a scab but inside a blood vessel.

blood count. Measurement of the number of red cells in the body. Red cells carry oxygen to the tissues.

bone marrow. Spongy material inside the bones. Produces the blood cells.

bone scan. A type of nuclear-medicine scan that allows a sensitive look at the entire skeleton for any changes that might suggest metastatic cancer.

bowel-prep. Cleansing of the intestines before abdominal surgery.

BPH (benign prostatic hyperplasia). Noncancerous enlargement of the prostate.

brachytherapy. Type of radiation treatment in which radioactive pellets are inserted into the prostate.

C

cancer. Abnormal and uncontrolled growth of cells in the body. Cancer can spread and ultimately injure and kill.

capsule. Fibrous outer lining of the prostate.

Casodex. Brand name for *bicalutamide*, an antiandrogen used to provide total androgen blockade.

castration. Removal of the testicles. See *orchiectomy*.

catheter. A hollow tube used to drain fluids from or inject fluids into body cavities.

cell. Smallest unit of the body. Cells make up tissues.

cell saver. Machine used to recycle blood lost during surgery and give it back to the patient during the procedure.

chemoprevention. Use of a substance to prevent the development and growth of cancer.

chemotherapy. Cancer treatment utilizing various powerful drugs to attack and destroy certain kinds of cancer.

clinical trials. Use of a new medication or treatment, under strict controls, to see if the new therapy is safe and effective.

colostomy. Surgical opening of the large intestine through the skin with drainage of the bowel contents into a bag.

complication. An undesirable result of a treatment, procedure or medication.

contracture. Scarring at the bladder neck after surgery, causing narrowing of the passage.

cryotherapy, cryosurgery. Freezing of the prostate for cancer therapy.

CT scan, CAT scan. A computerized X-ray of the body that shows the internal organs in cross-section view to visualize abnormalities. CT stands for *computerized tomography*. CAT stands for *computerized axial tomography*. The terms are synonymous.

cystoscope. Fiber-optic instrument used to look inside the bladder and urethra.

cystoscopy. Looking into the bladder or urethra under direct vision through a cystoscope.

D

DaVinci robotic laparoscopic prostatectomy. Use of the DaVinci three-dimensional robot to improve visualization and technique during laparoscopic prostatectomy.

debulk. To reduce the volume of cancer by surgery, hormone therapy or chemotherapy.

deep venous thrombosis. Formation of a clot in the large, deep veins, usually of the pelvis or legs.

deferred therapy. Delaying treatment until cancer becomes a definite threat to the patient.

DES (diethylstilbesterol). Type of female hormone, estrogen.

DHT (dihydrotestosterone). Active breakdown product of testosterone. DHT is more powerful than testosterone.

diagnosis. Determination of the cause or existence of a medical problem or disease.

diet. Regular eating and drinking habits. Specifically, what a person eats.

diethylstilbesterol (DES). Type of female hormone, estrogen.

digital rectal exam. Finger examination of the prostate gland through the rectum.

directed donations. Blood donated by friends or family for a patient with the hope it can be used if a transfusion is needed.

dissection. Surgical removal of tissue.

double-blind. Research study where neither doctor nor patient knows what medication or treatment is being used.

doubling time. Length of time for a set amount of cancer to double in size.

downsize. To shrink or reduce size of the cancerous tumor.

down-stage. To reduce the initial stage of a cancer to a lower and presumably better stage.

E

epidural anesthesia. Specific type of anesthesia in which a potent narcotic drips directly into the fluid that surrounds the spinal cord. This results in blockage of pain while allowing normal sensation and muscle function.

erectile dysfunction. Any abnormality in achieving or maintaining a penile erection.

estrogen. Female hormone.

estrogen therapy. Use of estrogen pills to block the male hormones as a treatment for advanced prostate cancer.

Eulexin. Brand name for flutamide, an antiandrogen used to provide total androgen blockade.

experimental. Untested or unproven treatment or approach.

external-beam therapy. The use of high-energy beams of radiation passed through tissues onto a target to kill rapidly growing cancer cells.

external vacuum device. A plastic tube used with suction to produce an erection. Used as a treatment for impotence.

F

family physician. Primary-care doctor who treats all members of a family.

fiber optics. New technology that allows looking at internal structures through fine fibers inside an instrument.

flutamide. A pill taken three times a day to provide total androgen blockade, blocking any remaining adrenal androgens from the cells. See *Eulexin.*

Foley catheter. Latex or silicone tube that drains urine from the bladder to an outside collecting bag.

frequency. Term to describe the need to urinate often.

frozen section. Preliminary rapid analysis of tissue by a pathologist who freezes the sample so a thin slice can be shaved off to use in microscopic examination. See also *permanent section.*

G

gatekeeper. Primary-care doctor, usually in an HMO, who controls referrals of patients to specialists for tests and evaluation.

general anesthesia. Total loss of consciousness or awareness prior to surgery because of medications.

genetics. Branch of science that studies heredity.

genitourinary tract. The urinary system (kidneys, ureters, bladder and urethra) and the genital system (testicles, vas deferens, prostate and penis).

gland. Structure or organ that produces a substance to be used in another part of the body.

grade. In cancer, the descriptive designation of the degree of malignancy based on the microscopic appearance of the cells.

groin. Part of the body where the legs attach to the torso on the lower abdomen.

gynecomastia. Enlargement of the male breast, often tender. Can occur on one side or both.

H

hematospermia. Blood in the semen.

hematuria. Blood in the urine.

heparin lock. A plug placed into an intravenous site that is periodically flushed.

heredity. Passing of characteristics from parents to children through genetic material.

hernia. Bulging of abdominal contents through a weakness in the abdominal wall, often in the groin.

hesitancy. Inability to start the urinary stream immediately.

high-grade. Very advanced cancer cells.

high-risk. More likely to have a complication or side effect.

HMO. Health maintenance organization.

hormones. Substances responsible for secondary sex characteristics.

hot flashes. Sudden feelings of heat, often with sweating and flushing of the skin, following hormone therapy.

hyperthermia. Heating of the prostate to destroy prostate tissue.

I

ICU. Intensive care unit. Section of hospital where critically ill patients or those requiring intensive observation and care are placed.

imaging. Seeing, through normal vision or X-rays.

immune system. Complicated system of organs, tissues, blood cells and substances that fight off infections, cancers or foreign proteins that can make you ill.

impotence. Inability to achieve and maintain an erection.

IMRT. Highly focused radiation technique.

incision. Cutting of the skin at the beginning of a surgical operation.

incontinence. Leaking of a substance. With urine, this is called *urinary incontinence*.

indications. Reasons for doing something.

inflammation. Swelling, pain, redness and irritation as a result of injury, surgery or infection.

informed consent. Permission given for a treatment by a person who is aware of the possible benefits as well as potential risks and complications.

inpatient. A person admitted to the hospital overnight.

internist. A type of primary-care physician who specializes in the nonsurgical management of disease and disease prevention.

interstitial. Within an organ, such as *interstitial radiation*, in which radioactive seeds are inserted into the prostate.

intravenous. Into the veins.

invasive. Moving beyond the organ of origin and into other tissues.

investigator. Doctor or scientist involved with an experimental study of a treatment or medication.

IVP (intravenous pyelogram). X-ray test using intravenous material that allows for visualization of the urinary tract.

K–L

Kegel exercises. Pelvic exercises that help to strengthen the muscles used with urination.

laparoscopy. Fiber-optic surgery performed through multiple, small incisions.

laser. Very powerful concentrated beam of high-energy light used in surgery.

LHRH analogue. Type of medication that causes the brain to stop stimulating testosterone production.

libido. Sex drive.

lifestyle. How a person chooses to live.

lobe. Either side of an organ, such as the prostate.

local anesthesia. Anesthesia or numbing of a specific area of the body.

local recurrence. Return of a cancer to the area where it was first located. See also *regional recurrence*.

localized. Contained or limited to the area described.

low-grade. Early stage of cancer-cell development.

Lupron. LHRH medication given as an injection every 28 to 84 days to drop testosterone levels for the treatment of advanced prostate cancer.

lycopene. Substance found in tomatoes that has powerful anticancer effects.

lymph. Clear fluid that bathes the cells of the body.

lymph-node dissection. Surgical removal of the lymph nodes that drain the prostate in the pelvis. Before the prostate gland is removed, nodes are examined microscopically to see if cancer is present.

lymph nodes. Small, bean-sized glands throughout the body that filter lymphatic fluid.

lymphadenectomy. Technical term for lymph-node dissection.

lymphangiography. An X-ray evaluation of the lymphatic vessels using a dye.

lymphocele. Collection or pocket of lymph fluid that has accumulated in the body.

M

malignancy. Uncontrolled growth of cells that can spread to other organs and cause death.

malignant. Cancerous, with the potential for uncontrolled growth and spread.

metastatic cancer. Cancer that has spread to other organs or tissues through the lymphatic or blood systems. (We say the cancer has *metastasized*.)

metastatic recurrence. The return of cancer in areas distant from the original cancer site.

microscopic. Small enough that a microscope is needed to see it.

moderately differentiated. Intermediate grade of cancer as determined by pathologic analysis of tissue.

MRI (magnetic resonance imaging). Tube-shaped device into which a person is placed for visualizing internal body structures. Not an X-ray.

N

negative. A test result that does not show what was being looked for.

neoadjuvant therapy. A treatment before surgery, such as radiation, hormone therapy or chemotherapy.

neoplastic. Malignant, cancerous.

nephrostomy tube. Small tube placed into the kidney through the skin that allows drainage of urine from the kidney.

Nilandron. Brand name for *nilutamide*, an antiandrogen used to provide total androgen blockade.

O

obturator nerve. A large nerve that travels in the pelvis and controls some leg movements.

oncologist. Specialized doctor who has taken several years of additional training after internal medicine and who deals with the evaluation and treatment of cancer.

orchiectomy. Surgical removal of the testicles.

organs. Tissues that work together for a specific function, such as bladder, heart or kidney.

outpatient. Describes a surgery or treatment that does not require an overnight stay in the hospital.

P

PAP. Prostatic acid phosphatase, a chemical once used to try to tell when prostate cancer had spread outside of the gland.

pathologist. Specially trained doctor who looks at tissues under a microscope to determine what they are and if disease is present. Pathologists also oversee laboratory tests such as the PSA blood test.

PCA3. Urine test to look for changes suggestive of prostate cancer.

pelvis. Part of the skeleton that forms a bony girdle joining the lower limbs of the body.

penile. Relating to the penis.

penile prosthesis. Surgically implanted device to provide erections for men who have become impotent, such as through prostate-cancer treatment.

perineal. Refers to an incision in the perineum to remove the prostate.

perineum. Area just behind the scrotum, in front of the anus.

permanent section. Formal preparation of tissue by a pathologist for microscopic analysis. See also *frozen section*.

PIN (prostatic intraductal neoplasia). An abnormal area seen on biopsied tissue. Is not cancerous but may become cancerous. May indicate that cancer is present in neighboring tissue.

placebo. Fake medication or treatment with no interaction with the body. Often used in research studies to test a new medication.

ploidy status. The genetic status of cancer cells; similar to the *grade*.

pneumatic sequential stockings. Inflatable stockings that squeeze the legs intermittently to help reduce the risks for serious blood clots.

poorly differentiated. High-grade, aggressive cancer, as determined by pathologic analysis of tissue.

positive biopsy. The detection of cancer in a biopsy.

positive margin. Condition in which cancer cells are found at the cut edge of tissue removed during surgery. A positive margin indicates that residual cancer may be remaining in the body.

posterior. Behind or toward the back.

prognosis. Act of foretelling the course of a disease. The long-term outlook or prospect for survival and recovery.

progression. Continued growth of the cancer or disease.

prostate. Gland located at the base of the bladder.

prostatectomy. Surgical removal of part or all of the prostate gland.

prosthesis. Artificial device used to replace the lost normal function of a structure or an organ.

protocol. Research study used to evaluate a specific treatment or medication.

proton-beam therapy. In conjunction with standard external-beam therapy, very powerful beams of protons are focused onto the prostate.

PSA (prostate specific antigen). Protein secreted by prostate cells, used to help detect and follow prostate cancer.

pulmonary embolus. Blood clot that travels along the large veins of the body up to the lungs. These can be instantly fatal if large enough.

R

radiation. Treatment utilizing X-rays to destroy cancerous tissues.

radiation therapist. Specially trained doctor who treats cancers with radiation therapy.

radical prostatectomy. Removal of the prostate gland and surrounding tissues and structures to eliminate cancer.

radioactive seeds. Small pellets of various substances that are treated to become radioactive, intended to kill adjacent cancer cells.

radiologist. Specially trained doctor who specializes in performing and interpreting various types of X-ray studies.

randomized. Term used in experimental studies to indicate treatment is randomly decided.

recovery room. Area in a hospital to which patients are transferred after surgery to recover before being sent to their rooms or homes, depending on the type of operation.

rectum. Last few inches of the intestine leading to the anus.

recurrence. Return of a disease.

refractory. Nonresponsive.

regional recurrence. Return of cancer in the same general area where it was first located. See also *local recurrence*.

regression. Shrinking of a tumor, either because of treatment or without obvious cause.

remission. Disappearance of the signs and symptoms of cancer. This can be temporary or permanent.

resectoscope. An instrument used to cut out prostate tissue through the urethra, under direct vision.

resistance. Ability to fight off a challenge. Some germs have developed a resistance to certain antibiotics. The body has a resistance to fighting infections.

retention. Inability to urinate.

retropubic. Behind the pubic bone.

risk. Chance or probability of something happening.

S

sampling error. In testing, when a problem exists but is not detected by the test.

scrotum. Sac that holds the testicles.

selenium. An element found in small amounts in food; may have anticancer effects.

semen. Fluid containing sperm that comes out of the penis during ejaculation.

seminal vesicles. Glands at the base of the bladder that add nutrients to the semen.

sepsis. Infection that causes high fever and shaking chills.

side effect. A secondary, usually adverse, reaction to a medication or treatment.

signs. Physical changes that can be observed by the patient or doctor. Signs occur as the result of a disease or disorder.

simulation. Technique using X-rays to plan radiation treatment for prostate cancer.

soy products. Products made from soybeans (a legume).

spasm. Rhythmic squeezing that can be painful, as with a bladder spasm.

spermine. Substance found in the prostate that slows the growth of prostate cancer.

sphincter. A bundle of muscles surrounding a tubular organ and controlling passage of fluids.

spinal anesthesia. Loss of sensation below the level of injection of medication on the spinal cord.

stage. Description of the size or quantity of a cancer and the extent of its spread from its original site.

stent. Tube that allows drainage from one place to another.

stricture. Scarring that squeezes a channel, such as the urethra.

suprapubic. Above the pubic bone, as in a *suprapubic incision* or *catheter*.

symptom. Condition that accompanies or results from a disease or disorder. The individual feels or experiences a symptom.

systemic. Throughout the body.

T

testicles. Two glands located inside the scrotum. They produce sperm, testosterone and other sex hormones.

testosterone. Primary male hormone.

therapy. Treatment for a disorder.

3-D conformal radiation therapy. Variation of standard external-beam therapy in which a computer, CT scan images and fitted brace are used to focus the radiation.

tissue. Specific type of material within the body, such as muscle, cartilage or hair.

total androgen blockade. Total blockage of all male hormones, using surgery and/or medications.

transferrin. Chemical in the body that has been shown to stimulate prostate cancer growth.

transperineal. Through the perineum, just under the scrotum and above the anus.

transrectal. Through the rectum.

transurethral. Through the urethra.

TRUS (transrectal ultrasound). Technique used to visualize the prostate and guide biopsies.

tumor. Abnormal tissue growth that can be cancerous (malignant) or noncancerous (benign).

tumor markers. Chemical substances that can be used to detect and follow the treatment of certain cancers.

tumor volume. Amount of cancer present in an organ.

TURP (transurethral resection of the prostate). Surgical technique performed under anesthesia through a fiberoptic instrument that is placed up the penis. Looking through the instrument, the physician can see prostate tissue that has grown and is blocking urinary flow through the urethra. This prostate tissue is removed with the instrument, leaving behind only the shell of the prostate.

U

undergrading. Term indicating that the grade of cancer is worse than that found in biopsied tissue.

ultrasound. A technique of visualizing internal organs by measuring reflected sound waves.

unit. Term referring to a pint of blood.

ureters. Muscular tubes that drain urine from the kidneys down to the bladder.

urethra. In men, the muscular tube that drains urine from the base of the bladder to the opening at the tip of the penis.

urgency. A sense of needing to urinate right away.

urinary retention. Inability to urinate, with the bladder filling up with urine.

urologist. Specially trained doctor who deals with the medical and surgical aspects of the genitourinary tract in men and women. This specialist deals with prostate cancer.

urostomy. A surgically made opening that enables urine to drain directly through the skin of the lower abdomen and then into a collection bag. This is performed when the bladder is removed.

V

vas deferens. Tiny tube that conveys sperm from the testicles to the prostate gland.

vasectomy. Minor operation to make a man sterile by cutting the vas deferens so that no sperm can pass through into the semen.

W

well-differentiated. Low-grade cancer as determined by pathologic analysis of tissue.

Z

Zoladex. LHRH medication in pellet form. It is inserted just under the skin to drop testosterone level for the treatment of advanced prostate cancer.

APPENDIX

Patient Information & Consent Forms

The following pages include printed materials that I give out from my office. They are similar to those you might receive from your doctor. They are included only for your information.

INSTRUCTIONS BEFORE PROSTATE ULTRASOUND & BIOPSY

To minimize the risks of infection and bleeding, we ask that you follow these instructions. If you have any questions or concerns, please call us. Our goal is to obtain the information necessary from the study while trying to make the experience as safe and comfortable as possible.

For most men, the procedure is uncomfortable. Though the potential serious problems are rare, following these guidelines significantly reduces any risks.

1. Avoid ASPIRIN or aspirin-containing products for TEN (10) days before the biopsy. You should also stop similar medications such as ibuprofen (Advil, Nuprin, Motrin, Anaprox) for THREE (3) days before the study. These medications can increase the risks for bleeding by interfering with normal clotting mechanisms. Tylenol (acetaminophen) is okay to take. If you have any questions about what should or should not be stopped, please call us.

2. Take a Fleets enema at home several hours before the biopsy. This can be obtained at any drug store.

3. Take an antibiotic, which we will prescribe, just as you leave your house to come to the office for the study. This will allow time for the medicine to be absorbed into your system and will reduce any chances of infection. At the time of the procedure you will also receive an antibiotic.

4. Though not absolutely necessary, having someone else drive you home is the best plan.

5. Following the study, you should plan to take it easy the rest of the day. You should avoid golf, swimming, tennis, traveling, etc. The next day

you may resume normal activities. Avoid alcohol until the following day, as well.

TRANSRECTAL ULTRASOUND AND BIOPSY OF THE PROSTATE

Transrectal ultrasound is a relatively new technique used to assist in the evaluation of the prostate. This technique allows visualization of the internal architecture of the gland, allowing identification and localization of any areas or lesions that may be suspicious for cancer. Using ultrasound guidance, prostate biopsies can now be obtained of areas that were previously not detected on simple rectal examination.

As in all aspects of medicine, this technique is not perfect. Some cancers will not be detected by ultrasound. This is why biopsies are performed even if no suspicious areas are identified, if there is reason to be suspicious. This way, by obtaining an adequate sampling of the prostate tissue, we can identify some cancers that might otherwise remain hidden.

This technique is performed in the office with a minimum of discomfort. No anesthesia is necessary. Using a high-speed biopsy device, several hairlike slivers of prostate tissue will be obtained and sent to a pathologist who specializes in the microscopic evaluation of tissue to determine if any cancer is present in the samples or if there are any other abnormalities.

Because cancer could be present but not seen on ultrasound or missed on biopsy (sampling error), it is important to follow up regardless of the biopsy results.

Prior to the study you should have taken an antibiotic tablet. At the time of the ultrasound, you will also receive an injection of a powerful antibiotic as well as several additional antibiotic pills to take following the biopsy: one pill twice a day until all are taken. This regimen will help to minimize the risk of infection in the urine, prostate or bloodstream.

Following the procedure, you may notice some blood in your urine, semen or bowel movements. This usually will pass within a few days but can persist off and on for up to a few weeks. Blood or discoloration can be seen in the semen occasionally up to a few months after the biopsy. Very rarely, some men will notice significant difficulty urinating after prostate ultrasound and biopsy. This can require a catheter to be placed, but usually only for a short time.

This procedure is usually very well tolerated. If you have any questions, please ask prior to beginning the procedure.

INSTRUCTIONS AFTER PROSTATE BIOPSY

The main risks following transrectal biopsy of the prostate include infection, bleeding and difficulty urinating. These guidelines should help minimize these risks and answer the most common questions and concerns. If you have any questions or problems, please do not hesitate to call at any time.

1. Take the antibiotics as directed: twice a day with a full glass of water until all are taken.
2. Blood in the urine, semen or bowel movements is common. This may be seen off and on for several days. You may also notice clots. There may be some blood or discoloration in the semen for several weeks or more.
3. There may be some burning or irritation with urination, which should last only a day or two.
4. Do not take aspirin or aspirin-containing products for several days after the biopsy, because this may increase the risk of bleeding.
5. After the biopsy, go home and take it easy the rest of the day. Tomorrow you may resume your normal activities.
6. Do not drink any alcohol until you have taken all of the antibiotics.
7. If you should experience a high fever, shaking, chills, severe abdominal or pelvic pain, heavy or prolonged bleeding, or difficulty or inability to urinate, please call me immediately. In the unlikely event you do not receive a prompt response and you feel that you are ill, go directly to the nearest emergency facility.
8. As soon as the pathology report is completed, I will notify you on the telephone. This can take from two to four days. If you have not heard from our office, please call us.

The following is a sample of a consent form to give you an idea of what you will be asked to sign. The one you are shown will undoubtedly be different.

Consent Procedure: Bilateral Pelvic Lymph-Node Dissection Radical Prostatectomy

I, (patient or guardian), authorize Dr._____, associates, and assistants of his/her choosing, to perform the following procedure: bilateral pelvic lymph-node dissection and radical retropubic prostatectomy. I understand the reason for the procedure is prostate cancer and the alternatives include observation, radiation or hormone therapy. If general anesthesia is required, the risks associated with my anesthesia should be discussed with my anesthesiologist.

In some cases the procedure may not be successful and I could be no better or even worse than I am now. For this reason, no guarantee can be given concerning the results. The result may be affected by complications that may occur.

This authorization is given with the understanding that any operation or procedure involves some risks and hazards. Some of the significant risks of this particular procedure include but are not limited to impotence, no ejaculation, incontinence, bladder-neck or urethral scarring, lymphatic fluid collection requiring additional surgery, nerve or blood-vessel injury, risk of transfusions, injury to adjacent organs including ureters, bladder, sphincter or rectum, risk for colostomy, and the possibility of residual or return of cancer requiring additional treatments.

I also understand that the more common risks of any procedure include infection, bleeding, nerve injury, blood clots, heart attack, allergic reactions, seizures, coma and pneumonia. These risks are serious and possibly fatal.

If you have any unanswered questions, please let us give you the answers prior to your signing this form.

Certification: I have read or had read to me the contents of this form and I understand the risks and alternatives involved regarding this procedure; I have had the opportunity to ask any questions I felt necessary, and all of my questions have been answered. I consent to the performance of this procedure.

(signed) _____

PROSTATE CANCER EVALUATION LOG

DATE / PSA / EXAM / BIOPSIES / PLAN FOR FOLLOW-UP

_____   _____

_____   _____

_____   _____

_____   _____

_____   _____

_____   _____

_____   _____

_____   _____

_____   _____

_____   _____

_____   _____

_____   _____

_____   _____

_____   _____

_____   _____

_____   _____

_____   _____

_____   _____

_____   _____

BIBLIOGRAPHY

American Cancer Society. National Conference on Prostate Cancer, Philadelphia, Pennsylvania, September/October 1994.

Bostwick, David G., M.D., MacLennan, G.T., M.D.; Larson, T.R. *Prostate Cancer, rev. ed.* American Cancer Society, 1999.

Gillenwater, Jay Y., M.D.; Grayhack, John T., M.D.; Howards, Stuart S., M.D.; Duckett, John W., M.D., editors. *Adult and Pediatric Urology.* Mosby Year Book, 1991.

Ginsberg, Beth, and Michael Milken. *The Taste for Living Cookbook: Mike Milken's Favorite Recipes for Fighting Cancer.* Time-Life, 1998.

Griffith, H. Winter, M.D. *Complete Guide to Prescription & Non-Prescription Drugs* (1998 ed.). Berkley Publishing Group, 1998.

Kirby, Roger, M.D.; Christmas, Timothy, M.D.; Brawer, Michael, M.D. *Prostate Cancer.* Times Mirror International Publishers, 1996.

McEvoy, Gerald K., Pharm.D., editor. *American Hospital Formulary Service Drug Information.* American Hospital Association, 2002.

Micozzi, Marc, M.D., Ph.D., editor. *Current Review of Complementary Medicine.* Current Medicine, 1999.

Morganstern, Steven, M.D.; Abrahams, Allen, Ph.D. *The Prostate Sourcebook: Everything You Need to Know, 3rd Ed.* Contemporary Books, 1998.

Moyad, Mark A. *The ABC's of Advanced Prostate Cancer.* Sleeping Bear Press, 2000.

Moyad, Mark A. *The ABC's of Nutrition & Supplements for Prostate Cancer.* Sleeping Bear Press, 2000.

Pilgrim, Aubrey. *A Revolutionary Approach to Prostate Cancer.* Sterling House, 1998.

Siegel, Mary-Ellen, M.S.W. *Dr. Greenberger's What Every Man Should Know About His Prostate.* Walker and Co., 1988.

Strum, Stephen B., and Donna Pogliano. *The Primer on Prostate Cancer: The Empowered Patient's Guide.* Life Extension Media, 2002.

Taguchi, Yosh, M.D. *Private Parts: An Owner's Guide to the Male Anatomy, 2nd ed.* McClelland & Stewart, 1996.

Walsh, Patrick, M.D., editor. *Campbell's Urology, 7th ed.* W.B. Saunders & Co., 1998.

Walsh, Patrick, M.D. *Guide to Surviving Prostate Cancer.* Warner Books, 2001.

INDEX

QUESTIONS AND NOTES FOR YOUR DOCTOR